PROFITS BEFORE PEOPLE?

Bioethics and the Humanities

Eric M. Meslin and Richard B. Miller, editors

LEONARD J. WEBER

PROFITS BEFORE PEOPLE?

ETHICAL STANDARDS AND THE MARKETING
OF PRESCRIPTION DRUGS

Indiana University Press

BLOOMINGTON AND INDIANAPOLIS

This book is a publication of

Indiana University Press
601 North Morton Street
Bloomington, IN 47404-3797 USA

http://iupress.indiana.edu

Telephone orders   800-842-6796
Fax orders   812-855-7931
Orders by e-mail   iuporder@indiana.edu

Library of Congress Cataloging-in-Publication Data

Weber, Leonard J., date
  Profits before people? : ethical standards and the
marketing of prescription drugs / Leonard J. Weber.
      p. ; cm. — (Bioethics and the humanities)
  Includes bibliographical references and index.
  ISBN 0-253-34748-3 (cloth : alk. paper)
  1. Pharmaceutical industry—Moral and ethical
aspects—United States. 2. Marketing—Moral and
ethical aspects—United States.
  [DNLM: 1. Drug Industry—ethics—United States.
2. Drug Industry—economics—United States.
3. Marketing—ethics—United States. 4. Pharmaceutical Preparations—United States. QV 736 W374p
2006] I. Title. II. Series.
  HD9666.5.W43 2006
  174'.96151—dc22   2005027198

1 2 3 4 5 11 10 09 08 07 06

To MMW

Contents

PART THREE

Acknowledgments

I am indebted to many individuals for supporting this project and for assistance in completing the manuscript, including Robert Hall, Carol Bayley, Michael McManus, Jessica Seck, Margaret Weber, and Gloria Albrecht. Thank you. I am particularly grateful to Thomas Schindler for repeated and careful review of the manuscript and for very helpful advice.

The School of Business at Gonzaga University provided the opportunity to begin to identify the issues addressed in this book by permitting me to teach a short course to MBA students on "Ethics and the Pharmaceutical Industry" while a Visiting Professor of Business Ethics in 2002–2004. The faculty "phased retirement program" at the University of Detroit Mercy made it possible for me to complete this project upon my return.

Working with different healthcare organizations as an ethics consultant has required that I apply ethical perspectives and analysis to a variety of issues and situations. In the process, I have learned that the most important contribution that an ethicist can make is to keep the focus on high ethical standards. I have attempted to apply that lesson here.

PROFITS BEFORE PEOPLE?

"It has all gone terribly wrong for the dozen or so manufacturers that make up 'big pharma.'" This statement introduced a review of the pharmaceutical industry's problems in a March 2005 article in *The Economist*.[1] The once well-respected drug companies are now being subjected to fierce criticism.

> They stand accused of focusing on "me-too" drugs which confer little clinical benefit over existing medicines; rushing these to market through cunning clinical trials designed to make them look better than they are; and suppressing data to the contrary. The industry is also lambasted for expensive, aggressive and misleading direct-to-consumer advertising, which sometimes creates conditions to fit the drugs, rather than the other way around.[2]

There is little trust that drug companies will do the right thing: a February 2005 Kaiser Family Foundation poll of 1,200 Americans found that 70 percent agreed that drug companies put profits ahead of people.[3]

When the pharmaceutical company Merck announced in the fall of 2004 that it was taking its blockbuster pain drug Vioxx (rofecoxib) off the market because of evidence that its use contributed to increased risks of heart attacks or strokes, some gave Merck credit for taking that action before it was mandated by the Food and Drug Administration (FDA). But many were not impressed by the company's overall Vioxx-related performance. There had been earlier warning signs of the risks associated with the use of Vioxx[4] and Merck's response at that time had been to continue to market the medication aggressively. By the time Merck made the decision to cease marketing Vioxx, millions of people were taking the drug, at a potential and unnecessary risk to their cardiovascular health. Vioxx was among the most heavily marketed, most widely used, and most profitable medicines, a case study of the way commercial interests can influence decisions about the marketing and use of drugs.

The FDA convened a panel of experts to advise on whether to permit the marketing of Vioxx and the other two painkillers in the class of drugs known as COX-2 inhibitors (Celebrex and Bextra). After the panel endorsed continued availability of these drugs, the Center for Science in the Public Interest did background checking and found that 10 of the 32 members of the advisory group had direct financial ties with the drug companies that make these drugs (received consulting fees, speaker fees, or research money from them).[5] "If the 10 advisors had not cast their votes, the committee would have voted 12 to 8 that Bextra should be withdrawn and 14 to 8 that Vioxx not return to the market. The 10 advisors with company ties voted 9 to 1 to keep Bextra on the market and 9 to 1 for Vioxx's return."[6] They were permitted to participate and vote despite the obvious questions about their objectivity. It is an important sign of the times that FDA panel reports are received with some skepticism precisely because of the potential influence of drug companies on these deliberations.

The pharmaceutical industry plays a key role in the American healthcare system and has had and continues to have an enormous influence on the practice of medicine. It sponsors much of the medical research being done; it produces the medicines that doctors prescribe and millions of people take; it sends out thousands of sales representatives to interact directly and frequently with physicians about the available drugs; it finances many of the continuing education programs physicians attend; it advertises drugs directly to the public, who are told to "ask your doctor" about the products; it contributes heavily to political campaigns and has a strong lobbying voice at the federal and state levels. It is a powerful industry whose practices affect the health and healthcare of many millions of people.

The pharmaceutical industry is now being subjected to criticism and challenge as never before in the age of scientific medicine. There has been increased critical attention paid to the methods that the industry uses to promote its products and to influence medical decisions. Much of the criticism is coming from physicians, often focused on the ways in which industry practices affect the quality of patient care and the professionalism and integrity of healthcare providers. The cost of prescription medications has been a major focus of concern among the public, one reflected in the debate about the provisions of the Medicare drug coverage legislation passed in 2003.

The number of recently published books critical of the pharmaceutical industry and of the general effects of commercialization on healthcare constitutes further evidence that a new era has begun.[7] The authors are generally well-respected and serious critics, most with long experience and impressive credentials. To cite three examples: Jerome Kassirer (*On the Take: How Medicine's Complicity with Big Business Can Endanger Your Health*) is a former editor in chief of *The New England Journal of Medicine;* Marcia Angell (*The Truth About the Drug Companies: How They Deceive Us and What to Do About It*) also held that position; Donald Barlett and James Steele (*Critical Condition: How Health Care in America Became Big Business—and Bad Medicine*) are Pulitzer Prize–winning journalists. Though the various books differ somewhat in their intent and in their selected points of focus, a common contention is that medical science and patient care suffer because of some of the ways in which businesses relate to practicing physicians, to medical researchers, to patients and the public, and to government and regulators.

The industry remains both wealthy and powerful, but the voices of the critics are getting stronger and louder. The message of the critics is clear: in the search for corporate profits, the drug industry, often with the complicity of medical professionals, engages in practices that can and frequently do lead to poor quality medical care and to treatment that is unnecessarily costly. The pharmaceutical industry contributes to important improvements in medical care, to be sure, but it also engages in practices that produce avoidable harmful effects. So say the critics.

These assessments of the role of the pharmaceutical industry help to identify practices that need systematic ethical analysis and reflection. Taking the critics seriously does not mean, of course, accepting their perspectives and/or their recommendations uncritically. They tell the kind of stories, though, that help to explain why it is necessary to establish and implement high ethical standards regarding such company practices as compensating physicians for serving as speakers or consultants, covering the cost of continuing medical education programs, providing incentives to physicians to enroll patients as subjects in clinical research projects, and advertising prescription drugs to the public through the mass media. The emerging critical literature is very helpful in identifying the issues that need more attention.

This book is a study of the place of commercial interests in marketing prescription drugs. For some, "marketing" simply means advertising; when they hear a comment about the marketing of prescription drugs, the first picture that comes to mind is the TV commercial that they just saw. For others, prescription drug "marketing" includes the visits of the sales representatives to doctors' offices. As used here, "marketing" includes these practices as well as many others. Companies market their products through all the ways in which they bring attention to their products, all the ways they spread the word about the benefits of their products, and all the ways that they establish relationships between themselves and the professionals who make treatment decisions. Accordingly, a study of drug marketing practices needs to include, in addition to advertising and visits by sales representatives, the industry's role in education, the provision of sample medications, even some clinical research practices. These are all methods that can be used to promote the use of a company's prescription drugs.

As a work of ethics, this book is not a descriptive study of the place of commercial interests in marketing prescription drugs. It is, rather, an effort to understand the proper place of commercial interests in marketing prescription drugs. A major part of the ethicist's task is to clarify the nature of the relevant responsibilities and to help identify good ethical practices regarding the identified issues. The ultimate goal is to assist in answering the practical ethics question ("What is the right or best thing to do in these circumstances, all relevant responsibilities considered?"). Both the perspectives of the critics and the guidelines that the industry itself has adopted have made some contributions here, but much more needs to be done. The lack of confidence in the pharmaceutical industry is, fundamentally, a doubt about the industry's ethics: a concern that the drug companies are engaged in practices that represent the wrong priorities; a conviction that big pharma is failing to understand its basic responsibilities.

Ethics and the law are clearly not the same. What is legally permissible is not always an ethically acceptable business practice. Lynn Sharp Paine has put it this way: "Our system of government guarantees us rights that it may be unethical to exercise on certain occasions. Terminology may make it easy to lose sight of the distinction between 'having a right' and 'the right thing to do,' but the distinction is critical."[8] Taking ethics seriously means recognizing that the law does not answer all questions about what is right. Law may establish the ethical minimum, but the most important ethical judgments often need to be made in a context of legal permissibility. What should we do when we can take different approaches, all of which are legally acceptable? One legally permissible way of marketing pharmaceuticals may well be considerably more appropriate, all relevant ethical responsibilities considered, than another legally permissible way. The analysis and reflection involved in "doing ethics" are intended to lead to the identification of the right or best practice and the reasons for concluding that one course of action is the right or best practice. The fact that the law does not prohibit a particular industry practice is not a reasonable basis either for engaging in it or for defending it.

Business ethics is not primarily about individual behavior. In seeking to implement high ethical standards for marketing prescription drugs, the focus of attention here is not on the behavior of an individual sales representative or of a symposium speaker. It is more important to consider industry-wide practices, practices that may be, in fact, quite widely accepted as standard or appropriate. Given the nature and impact of this particular industry and the potential consequences of a particular marketing-related practice, does this practice reflect high ethical standards? Sustained and focused consideration on the relevant responsibilities just might point the way to more demanding ethics standards and better practices. And this, in turn, might begin to restore some confidence in the drug industry.

Despite its central role in healthcare, the pharmaceutical industry has not yet received much systematic attention in deliberations on healthcare ethics. Much more attention has been given to issues involved in the clinical provision of healthcare than to the issues involved in the business side of healthcare. This is beginning to change, but there is not yet a well-developed understanding of the demands of good healthcare business ethics. Neither healthcare professionals nor the public are very clear yet on how to draw the line between ethically acceptable and unacceptable practices in businesses providing healthcare services or products. And not one of the recent books on the pharmaceutical industry was explicitly framed as an ethics project.[9] This one is.

The pharmaceutical industry is a for-profit industry. One essential part of the task of clarifying the ethical standards to which the industry should be held accountable in its marketing practices is, therefore, a review of the ethical responsibilities of for-profit business. In a discussion of the relationship of physicians to drug companies, David Blumenthal included the following comment: "As a for-profit business, the pharmaceutical industry should be expected to market its products aggressively within legal boundaries."[10] In the context in which the statement is found, it seems clear that to market "aggressively" means to use enticements and to provide selective information on the benefits and risks of a company's drugs. It means company practices that can result in conflicts of interest for physicians and that might contribute to their having an incomplete understanding of the effects of the medications. It is less clear, though, what Blumenthal means by the phrase "should be expected." It might mean that, because for-profit companies sometimes act this way driven by their commercial interests, we should be prepared for the pharmaceutical industry to act this way. Or "should be expected" might mean that the industry should act in this way, that it is right that they do so. These are two very different meanings. The first is a recognition that the profit motive can be a very powerful incentive, so powerful that it can, at times, distort a company's understanding of its true ethical responsibilities. We should be prepared for pharmaceutical companies doing whatever is legal to sell their products because, under pressure to show high profits, they do not always engage in good ethical practices. According to the second meaning, always putting profits first and foremost (within legal boundaries) is, in fact, the ethical responsibility of for-profit business. In this understanding of ethics, pharmaceutical companies are acting properly in doing whatever is legal to sell their products, even when it might compromise the integrity of healthcare professionals and the quality of medical care. Given the world of difference between these two approaches to business ethics, it is essential to begin the reflections on appropriate ethics standards for the pharmaceutical industry by considering the right relationship between ethics and profit.

The first section of the book presents a framework for understanding the general ethical responsibilities of pharmaceutical companies, as for-profit businesses and as pharmaceutical companies. The following two sections divide the issues and concerns related to marketing prescriptions drugs between those raised by marketing to healthcare professionals and those raised by marketing to the public. In each case, the section begins with an effort to provide and explain the ethical vision and framework that informs the analysis of specific issues and that leads to the judgments that are made. A work of this sort requires a willingness on the part of the author to advocate a point of view and to take stands. Any one person's understanding and sensitivity are, of course, always limited and incomplete. Nevertheless, the effort to identify ethical standards that apply to the practices under consideration might assist others who are also seeking to clarify the limits of commercial interests as the pharmaceutical industry markets its products.

The critics have concluded that the pharmaceutical industry has gone terribly awry. In Angell's words: "Now primarily a marketing machine to sell drugs of dubious benefit, this industry uses its wealth and power to co-opt every institution that might stand in its way, including the U. S. Congress, the Food and Drug Administration, academic medical centers, and the medical profession itself."[11] The prescription drug industry is now being challenged to reform itself and the public is being challenged to insist that it is reformed. The purpose of this book is to consider the kinds of concerns and standards and marketing-related practices that the public can legitimately demand that the industry adopt, ones that reflect an acceptable balance between commercial interests and the needs of healthcare professionals, of patients, and of the public.

PART ONE

THE LIMITS OF COMMERCIAL INTERESTS

1

Ethics and For-Profit Business

Knowing how to relate ethics and the financial bottom line is one of the biggest challenges facing all who seek to manage a business responsibly. Neither ethics education nor business education has, it appears, adequately prepared most people to include dollars comfortably and skillfully in ethical discernment and to include ethics comfortably and skillfully in cost and revenue considerations. It can be extraordinarily difficult to decide how best to reconcile or balance concern for the financial impact on the organization of a particular policy or practice with concern for other considerations about the "rightness" of that policy or practice.

This has certainly been the case in healthcare ethics. The emphasis until recently has been primarily on individual patient care. A typical "case consultation" in medical ethics is a request for assistance in deciding what to do in regard to the treatment of a critically ill or dying patient. Discussion usually focuses on the physician's judgment regarding reasonable treatment options and on the patient's expressed beliefs about acceptable and unacceptable treatment, if these beliefs are known. The consultation may also address whatever other concerns are raised by the patient's family or by other professionals involved in the care of the patient. Almost never do the cost of the treatment and the implications of that cost for the family, the payer, the provider, or the healthcare system receive careful and detailed analysis. The cost questions are, in all probability, on the minds of some involved in the deliberations, but there is either a sense that it is inappropriate to take cost into account when making decisions about medical ethics or, if judged appropriate, there is little confidence about how to explore sensitively the ethical relevance of the cost.

Though the above description remains true of the typical ethics case consultation in America's hospitals, the field of healthcare ethics is beginning to change. The last few years have seen much more attention given to "organizational ethics," to ethical issues facing management in healthcare. While many clinicians remain committed to thinking about only one patient at a time and remain wary of considering money when deciding what is best for that patient, managers tend to recognize that it would be irresponsible not to consider the financial impact of their decisions. Bottom-line sensitivity is an ethical responsibility, not just a practical necessity.

Expanding the focus of ethical concerns beyond the bedside is leading to the recognition that knowing what is "the right thing to do" in healthcare means taking financial impact into account, in addition to the other considerations. Attending to the bottom line is an ethical responsibility, but it is not the only one. It is not easy to know when financial considerations should take priority over other considerations in a healthcare organization—and when they should not take priority—and it is the on-going task of ethicists to provide some guidance.

Contrary to what often happens in medicine, there has never been reluctance in business to emphasize the importance of the bottom line. While there has been a tendency among some healthcare professionals to make decisions that play down or ignore the significance of "money," business appears to play down or ignore the significance of "ethics." Over the years, companies have usually been evaluated as successful or not based on their profitability and their attractiveness to investors, not on their reputation for ethics. When challenged on practices critics thought harmful to the public, a common response in past decades was to insist that "the business of business is business." The role of business in society, it was argued, is to focus on the bottom line and not to be concerned about the implications for society, as long as nothing illegal is done.

For a number of years, when meeting new people and responding to the question of what kind of work I do, I have said that, among other things, I teach business ethics. This has gotten interesting and, after a while, predictable responses. Two common one-line responses have been "Business ethics: isn't that an oxymoron, a contradiction in terms?" and "That must be a very short course!" Though these comments are intended to be humorous, they seem to reflect a widespread perception that "business" and "ethics" are commonly at odds, that one cannot really expect business to adhere to high ethical standards. The perception that for-profit businesses are driven solely by a concern for profit and/or the value of their stock is an understandable point of view. The Enron and WorldCom cases, among others, have reminded all of us that company management does not always feel restricted even by the law in their pursuit of profit or shareholder wealth or "success."

An ABC special with Peter Jennings, *Bitter Medicine: Pills, Profit and the Public Health,* broadcast in May 2002, included an interview that Jennings did with Drummond Rennie, an editor of *JAMA: the Journal of the American Medical Association.* Jennings asked Dr. Rennie whether he believed that drug companies "are intent on keeping consumers on drugs, which are not as good as older drugs, for the simple requirement of profit." Rennie responded yes, absolutely, and it would be strange if they didn't. "They've got to be prevented."[2] Rennie's point was that the pharmaceutical industry needs to be understood as part of the for-profit business world. And he understood this to mean that such businesses will do whatever they can in the pursuit of profits, even if their activities interfere with the practice of good medicine, and that the only way to prevent them is by legal restraints.

The perception that business cannot be expected to be seriously committed to interests other than profit is understandable, but it does not reflect contemporary business philosophy. During the last two decades or so, it has become increasingly common for business leaders to acknowledge additional concerns and responsibilities besides making profit and observing the law. Today one rarely hears the comment that "the business of business is business." Instead, it has become common in recent years for business executives to make the claim that "good ethics is good business." The expressed commitment to taking ethics seriously is the present frame of reference for any discussion of the responsibilities of businesses. It invites the public to expect and demand that for-profit businesses recognize other ethical and social responsibilities beyond those to owners/shareholders and beyond the minimum ethical standards imposed by law.

GOOD ETHICS IS GOOD BUSINESS

The healthcare system includes both service or charitable organizations and business enterprises. Whether it is desirable to have for-profit industry occupy key roles in the healthcare system is a legitimate question, one that deserves additional attention, but it is not the focus of this study. Rather, the intent here is to consider the ethical responsibilities of for-profit businesses (first in general and later with a specific focus on the pharmaceutical industry). There is a difference between for-profit and not-for-profit organizations, to be sure, but for-profit businesses also have other responsibilities in addition to profit making.

As a result of what is sometimes referred to as "the business ethics movement,"[3] it has become increasingly clear that companies have an ethical responsibility to take into account the impact of their practices, policies, and decisions on all those affected (all stakeholders) and to find the proper balance among the benefits and burdens distributed among different stakeholder groups. Shareholders or owners are one important stakeholder group, but they are not the only one. Dr. Rennie's comment is understandable in the context of his experiences and concerns, but it is not at all "strange" to expect that at times for-profit companies put other considerations before profit. In many situations, it is exactly what corporate executives should do and what the public should insist they do.

Kenneth Mason, former president of Quaker Oats, is reported to have said: "Making a profit is no more the purpose of a corporation than getting enough to eat is the purpose of life." Getting enough to eat is necessary for life, but "life's purpose, one would hope, is somewhat broader and more challenging."[4] For Mason and for many others, profit is seen as an essential means to achieving the real purpose of business: meeting the needs of society by providing valuable goods or services. Being "for-profit" implies that profit is central, clearly more central than in not-for-profit service organizations, but being for-profit does not mean that profit is the only important responsibility of the business. It is of interest to read the mission, vision, and value statements of different companies. Profit or superior rate of return for investors is commonly included in a company's stated understanding of what it is about, but it is not the only claim made about the mission.

Many business executives, business consultants, and business critics agree with the claim that "good ethics is good business." This statement is open to different interpretations, but for most who make such a claim it means that following high ethical standards is related to—and contributes to—business success. It is even becoming common to claim that profit-seeking and a commitment to the public good go hand-in-hand: "We share a strong belief, backed by growing empirical evidence, that tomorrow's most successful and competitive companies will be those that combine a commitment to profitability with an explicit commitment to advancing the public interest."[5] The claim or belief is that ethics puts a company at a competitive advantage, that ethics pays. Good ethics contributes to business success in that high ethical standards encourage trust in the company and improve the company's reputation. Some executives are recognizing that "a reputation for ethical and socially responsible behavior can be the basis for a 'competitive edge' in both market and public policy relationships."[6] On the other hand, behavior that results in conflict and suspicion reduces the likelihood of business success.

This could well be true—sometimes. A commitment to a high standard of ethics probably does lead to bottom-line success at times. But ethics does not guarantee high profits and cannot be expected to contribute to profits in every case. Nor is it true to imply that ignoring ethical responsibilities is always unprofitable. High profits are not necessarily a sign of good ethics. The claim that "good ethics is good business" may be a misleading description of the impact or the consequences of a commitment to ethics.

The traditional way of speaking about the profit-making goal is in terms of "maximum profits" or profit maximization. It may be more compatible with an understanding of other responsibilities in addition to profit to speak of "optimum profits." "Maximum." means the most, the greatest possible. "Optimum" means the best, the most suitable. The pursuit of "maximum profits" carries with it the very real risk of ignoring or overriding all other responsibilities. The pursuit of "optimum profits" appears more open to recognizing the relevance and importance of other considerations.

A belief that good ethics is good business may actually undermine a true commitment to ethics. W. Michael Hoffman's observation is worth noting:

> One thing the study of ethics has taught us over the past 2500 years is that being ethical may on occasion require that we place the interests of others ahead of or at least on par with our own interests. And this implies that the ethical thing to do, the morally right thing, may not be in our own self-interest. . . . We should promote business ethics, not because good ethics is good business, but because we are morally required to adopt the moral point of view in all our dealings, and business is no exception. In business, as in all human endeavors, we must be prepared to pay the cost of ethical behavior.[7]

If it is expected that good ethics and business success routinely go hand in hand, we could be tempted at times to consider practices to be good ethics if (or only if) they lead to business success. Since we are all capable of the kind of self-deception that identifies our own personal or organizational self-interest with the public good, it is important to be wary of claims (like "good ethics is good business") that might encourage us to do just that.

Still, while there are reasons not to endorse the understanding that "ethics pays," the statement that "good ethics is good business" can be understood in a way that can be fully supported. It is good business to take ethics seriously, to be committed to excellence in ethics. This is good business because it reflects a proper understanding of what is owed to the public and to other stakeholders. A practice or a decision is good business if and only if it is good ethics—if it reflects the appropriate understanding of responsibilities to all stakeholders. As is indicated in the quote from Hoffman, business is no exception to the general expectation that we be ethical in all our endeavors. It is not always easy to know what is the ethically right thing to do in particular business situations, but what can be expected and demanded of any business is a commitment to taking ethics seriously, to seeking to know and do the right thing. Unless that commitment is present, a business can hardly be described as a good business.

A COMMITMENT TO BUSINESS ETHICS

It is one thing to state a commitment to good ethics; it is something else to live out such a commitment. Good ethics is not easy. It is difficult to do the right thing when that involves some unwanted cost. It is also difficult, many times, to understand what the right thing to do is in particular circumstances. Different persons, with similar commitments to ethics, might well disagree about what good ethics means in specific situations. This fact does not mean that one answer is as good as another. Rather, it means that all involved need to be willing to engage in the efforts necessary to apply the best understanding of the ethical significance of the issue to the present situation. The hard work of ethics requires careful and ethically sensitive examination of specific issues.

It may be useful to review a few of the general implications of what it means for companies to take business ethics seriously.

A commitment to good business ethics means recognizing that ethics is about more than observing all applicable laws and regulations.

Ethical responsibility includes observing laws and regulations, but it is not limited to that. Not everything legally permissible is good ethical practice. As noted in the introduction, many of the ethical issues that merit the most attention of business leaders and the public are ones that cannot be answered by legal analysis. Lynn Sharp Paine puts it this way in a discussion of advertising to young children: "Even if advertisers have a constitutional right to advertise lawful products to young children in a nondeceptive way, it is not necessarily the right thing to do. Our system of government guarantees us rights that it may be unethical to exercise on certain occasions."[8] The most challenging ethical issues for business commonly involve determining what course of action to take among legally permissible options. Obviously, the best answer is not determined solely by knowing what is legally permitted.

There is an additional point to be made here. When members of the public make ethical demands of a company—when they say that the company "should" or "should not" do something—they are not necessarily saying that their position should be imposed by law. Frequently, they are seeking to get the company to acknowledge and voluntarily act on a specific understanding of what is the right thing to do in the circumstances. They are more likely to seek public policy changes if they believe that legal mandates are the only way to bring about changes in industry or company practices.

A commitment to good business ethics means recognizing that ethics is about more than the behavior of individuals. It is at least as much about the policies and practices of the company.

One common expression of a company's commitment to ethics is a code of ethics or a code of conduct for employees. In their employee codes of ethics, companies not only insist that it is important to do the right thing, but they also often go into considerable detail in clarifying for employees what is the right thing to do in a variety of circumstances. These codes, especially when combined with an effective ethics education program, provide useful clarification and guidance regarding expected behaviors and are an important part of promoting ethics in the workplace.

In recent years, a significant number of companies have established an ethics office and/or have appointed an ethics officer. In addition to responsibility for providing education on the code, individuals in these positions often manage a "hotline" for questions about appropriate behavior and for employee reports about possible wrongdoing. The ethics officer's attention is usually focused on compliance with legal mandates as well as with a company's own internal ethics policies. This can contribute to the mistaken identification of the ethical with the legally permissible.

Given the emphasis on employee codes of ethics, as well as the general tendency in American society to identify any question of ethics with individual behavior, it is not surprising that many think of business ethics as being about the behavior of individuals in the workplace. Business ethics does include consideration of individual behavior (what it means to be an ethical businessperson), but it is also concerned with the policies and practices of a company (what it means to be an ethical company). In fact, more people are likely to be affected in more serious ways by company policies and practices than by the behavior of individuals acting as individuals—for example, by decisions about employee wages and benefits, by the selection of particular advertising techniques to promote a product, or by the policy chosen on acceptable environmental risk. These are company practices or policies and not simply decisions made by individuals based on their own personal moral values, though individuals can, of course, contribute to the decision-making that determines the policies and practices.

The practical ethics question (what is the right thing to do in the circumstances, all relevant responsibilities considered) needs to be consistently asked and answered, regardless of whether the context is individual behavior or company policy.

A commitment to good business ethics means understanding that how well a company is meeting its ethical responsibilities is determined by what it does, not by what it says or what image it presents.

There is often the tendency or temptation, when considering ethics, to want to make ourselves look good. We want to be perceived as meeting responsibilities and adhering to high ethical standards, as individuals and as leaders of organizations. The tendency is to emphasize our goodwill, our integrity, and our commitment to social responsibility. When a company practice or policy is challenged, the temptation is to "manage the issue" by using all the marketing and public relations techniques and skills available to make the company look good. A true commitment to ethics means focusing on public responsibility, not just public image.

Business ethics requires that we hold ourselves and others accountable for meeting the full range of responsibilities. It requires that attention be placed on actions and their consequences, more than on intentions and on interpretations given to what is happening. As is discussed later, the practical ethical responsibilities of a business are often best understood through stakeholder analysis—determining who is being affected and in what ways by company decisions and practices. Goodwill and good intentions are important, but they do not guarantee awareness of or attention to the implications of actions for different stakeholders or insight into the significance of these implications. Nor do they automatically mean an understanding of the appropriate priorities among various responsibilities.

A commitment to good business ethics means that, to the greatest extent possible, company executives should not take a criticism of their company's policies or practices as the same thing as a criticism of their personal integrity.

When a company or industry is being criticized for a particular practice or for its approach to a particular issue, industry/company leaders should not take this as an accusation that they are personally unethical or that they are insufficiently interested in ethical considerations. Disagreements about what is the right thing to do in specific circumstances are usually best approached as a difference of opinion about ethical responsibilities. It is often a difference in understanding the role and function of business in society. Different people, all sincerely seeking to adhere to high ethical standards, might well disagree about what is the right thing to do. If members of the public challenge a company's practice, they are best understood as saying the company is misunderstanding its responsibilities or has misplaced priorities. It may be difficult for company leaders not to feel that their personal ethics are being criticized when a company practice is challenged as irresponsible, but it is important to try to keep the focus on the question of what the company should be doing rather than on whether an individual is being identified as a "bad person."

Good ethics is hard work. In addition to wanting to do what is right, a commitment to ethics often requires listening to and consulting with others in order to discern what is right in the particular circumstances. A commitment to high ethical standards needs to include a willingness to listen to those who disagree and a desire to learn from others. We all, as individuals and as companies or industries, have a tendency to analyze issues from our own limited perspective. Getting a view of the whole picture almost always requires contributions from others. A defensive response to criticism may be natural, but it does not further the goal of achieving good business ethics.

A commitment to good business ethics means understanding that social responsibility is not primarily about philanthropy. It is first and foremost about the benefits and harms to relevant stakeholders resulting from the day-to-day business of the company.

Many corporations today speak of their "social responsibility" as part of their effort to be good corporate citizens. Increasingly, they are issuing reports on their efforts and plans related to social and environmental issues, recognizing that the public is interested in the social and environmental impact as well as in the financial record (the three are sometimes referred to as "the triple bottom line"). Being socially and environmentally responsible is a major part of what it means to be committed to good ethics.

Sometimes a company will describe its social responsibility in terms of the philanthropic contributions made—such as donations to education or charities and released time for workers to serve as volunteers. While these are almost always welcomed by the communities served, they are not at the heart of a business or its role in society. Philanthropy should be considered as something over and above what the public can legitimately demand. The public should demand that every business conduct its regular activities in ways that are compatible with its responsibilities to benefit stakeholders and to avoid significant harm to society or the environment. The "private" nature of business means that solving social problems (those that they did not create or exacerbate) is not at the heart of what they owe the public. But it does not mean that business has no duty to society.

Philanthropy is a work of charity. It is fine if a business wants to make philanthropic contributions, but such contributions are not essential for a business to be a good business. What is essential is that a business meets its obligations to the public, doing what is owed to different stakeholders or constituencies. A company that makes major philanthropic contributions but, for example, has a questionable record in regard to avoiding or restricting the harm done by its regular business activities, has clearly not grasped the essence of social responsibility.

> *A commitment to good business ethics means recognizing that specific ethical responsibilities are largely determined by the nature of the industry or business.*

This chapter began with the following statement from Jay Cohen: "No one expects business enterprises to act like charitable organizations. However, we do expect companies to draw the line when their policies cause harm."[9] This is the very minimum. For those companies that provide optional or non-essential products or services, the emphasis can be placed on the need to avoid causing harm (to employees, customers, the community, etc.) in the pursuit of private interests. Businesses, on the other hand, whose products and/or services are necessary or very important for the public good, have a higher level of responsibility. In addition to avoiding harm, they need to provide the kind of quality product or service needed at a price that is affordable. Healthcare businesses, including pharmaceutical companies, provide products or services that are often needed for a good quality of life. Even when these organizations are private, for-profit, they owe the public more than simply avoiding causing harm. Not all for-profits are the same.

> *A commitment to good business ethics means learning some tools (key concepts, guiding principles) and understanding the process (application of guiding principles to specific situations) involved in making practical ethical judgments.*

As noted above, good ethics is not easy. It involves knowledge and skill as well as personal integrity. Without ethical integrity, there is not an incentive to seek to know and do the right thing. But integrity among business leaders is not sufficient by itself. Unless they are also educated in recognizing and balancing the range of stakeholder responsibilities, persons of integrity will not have the necessary insight into what is at stake in business policies and practices. Unless they are also skilled in translating general responsibilities to particular situations, persons of integrity will not be able to move from good intentions to good practice. Good ethics practices result from effort: study, consultation, and listening to key stakeholders are often necessary.

THE NEED FOR A WATCHFUL PUBLIC

Profit-seeking and ethics are compatible; it is not an oxymoron to bring together "business" and "ethics." Identifying a for-profit business as an organization that pursues only the goal of financial success (within the restraints imposed by law) does not promote high ethical standards. Expecting companies to be one-dimensional, limiting their ethical responsibilities to profit maximization, may encourage them to do just that.

On the other hand, it is also important that the public be somewhat skeptical about a stated commitment of business to ethics and to social responsibility. Corporate claims about the importance of ethics can be sincere, but they can also be a public relations effort to polish the company's image. Even when sincere, the words may not be reflected in the company's practices. Even when the claim is sincere, the understanding of ethical responsibilities may be much too narrow and limited. Companies, including the best companies, need to be challenged to show results in practice.

There is a constant temptation in business to allow profit-making goals to trump other responsibilities that are, in the bigger picture, of greater importance or higher priority. Business executives do not need to be reminded of the importance of profit. Wall Street, their own training, and reward systems will ensure that the importance of profit will not be ignored. The business system, however, does not have built into it the same sort of guarantee that all other important responsibilities will receive management's full attention. The pressure to keep responsibilities in proper perspective often needs to come from the outside. The public has an essential role to play in insisting that companies keep priorities straight.

[P]rescription drugs are not like ordinary
goods, and the market for drugs is not like
other markets. The misconception that drugs
and their market are like other goods and
markets explains most of the serious problems
with the pharmaceutical industry today.[1]

2

The Pharmaceutical Industry

and Its Stakeholders

One of the most important developments in business ethics in
recent years has been recognizing the importance of stakeholder
analysis in determining ethical responsibility. "Stakeholders" are
identified as those who have something at stake in a company's
"products, operations, markets, industry, and outcomes."[2] They
are "persons and groups that stand to benefit from, or be harmed
by, corporate activity."[3] Stakeholders include, first of all, those
who have entered into a voluntary association with the company
and are, therefore, directly affected by the ways that company does
its business. Examples are investors, employees, customers, and
suppliers. But stakeholders also include many who have not voluntarily associated themselves with the company at all, but who
are nonetheless affected by company practices, such as those who
are part of the local community in which the business is located
or those who are exposed to a company's mass media advertising
of its products.

The term "stakeholder" is obviously contrasted with "stock-holder" and is useful in emphasizing the inadequacy of a philosophy which holds that a company's only responsibility is to protect and promote the interests of stockholders or owners. Companies have a responsibility to various constituencies, not just to one. Any serious effort to understand a particular company's responsibility requires sustained attention to the ways that various stakeholders are affected by the company's practices and a recognition of what is owed to the different stakeholders. It requires, as well, an understanding of how best to balance the different stakeholder needs and interests when they cannot all be met or satisfied.

In using a stakeholder approach, it is essential to consider the specific nature of an industry in order to address practical questions of business ethics. Different industries are engaged in different kinds of business and, as such, have different types of effects on different stakeholders. Some industries are more central to meeting the basic needs of the public, a fact that has important implications for the kind of demands that the public can appropriately make of that industry. The stakeholders in one industry may have different vulnerabilities and may be exposed to different risks of harm than those in another industry. Medicines are different from automobiles, from clothes, from pesticides, from computers, from restaurant meals. Given the different issues involved in different industries, it is not sufficient to reflect only upon generic concerns in business ethics or marketing ethics. Good ethics requires attention to industry-specific considerations.

WHAT ALL BUSINESSES OWE STAKEHOLDERS

In 1999, a group of scholars published the results of a collective effort to identity principles that can be used to understand a corporation's responsibilities to stakeholders. These "Principles of Stakeholder Management" are a good starting point for taking stakeholders seriously. Published by the Clarkson Centre for Business Ethics at the University of Toronto, the principles are often referred to as the "Clarkson Principles."

PRINCIPLES OF STAKEHOLDER MANAGEMENT

PRINCIPLE 1   Managers should *acknowledge* and actively *monitor* the concerns of all legitimate stakeholders, and should take their interests appropriately into account in decision-making and operations.

PRINCIPLE 2   Managers should *listen* to and openly *communicate* with stakeholders about their respective concerns and contributions, and about the risks that they assume because of their involvement with the corporation.

PRINCIPLE 3   Managers should *adopt* processes and modes of behavior that are sensitive to the concerns and capabilities of each stakeholder constituency.

PRINCIPLE 4   Managers should *recognize the interdependence* of efforts and rewards among stakeholders, and should attempt to achieve a fair distribution of the benefits and burdens of corporate activity among them, taking into account their respective risks and vulnerabilities.

PRINCIPLE 5   Managers should *work cooperatively* with other entities, both public and private, to insure that risks and harms arising from corporate activities are minimized and, where they cannot be avoided, appropriately compensated.

PRINCIPLE 6   Managers should *avoid altogether* activities that might jeopardize inalienable human rights (e.g., the right to life) or give rise to risks which, if clearly understood, would be patently unacceptable to relevant stakeholders.

PRINCIPLE 7   Managers should *acknowledge the potential conflicts* between (a) their own role as corporate stakeholders, and (b) their legal and moral responsibilities for the interests of stakeholders, and should address such conflicts through open communication, appropriate reporting and incentive systems and, where necessary, third party review.[4]

The Clarkson Principles serve as a basis for considering the responsibilities of all companies to their stakeholders.

In order to take stakeholder concerns into account, management needs to know what these concerns are, especially how different stakeholders stand to benefit from or be harmed by company practices.

One of the most difficult challenges facing a firm's management is the need to know, in a realistic way, the implications for various stakeholders of company practices. Some concerns are evident. Stock market prices allow management to make a reasonable judgment about the return-on-investment interests of many stockholders. When shareholder resolutions are submitted, they clearly express the concerns of those who file them. Purchases of products reveal something about customer interests, just as liability lawsuits or boycotts reveal specific concerns. Other stakeholder concerns are less easy to ascertain. The information that companies routinely track may not provide much insight, for example, into the concerns of informed citizens about the impact of company practices on the environmental health of the local community.

As an organization that is part of the larger society and has an impact on both voluntary and involuntary stakeholders, a business has a minimum responsibility to avoid doing harm to these stakeholders. This requires a clear awareness of the risks to which various constituencies are exposed because of company policies and practices. In many cases, these risks are not immediately known; indeed, they are not easily recognized even by those affected. The effect of plant discharges on the quality of the water or air may not be immediately evident, at least to a typical citizen. The same can be said about the consequences of programming TV entertainment containing violence during children's viewing hours.

Taking stakeholders seriously often means, therefore, listening to public interest groups and other activists (especially those who have done research) who are expressing concerns related to some company or industry practices. Critics, however unwelcome they might be to managers who are conscientiously trying to do their jobs well, are an important source of information about possible risks to which a company is exposing stakeholders. Listening to stakeholders carefully often means taking critics seriously.

The purpose of listening to critics is to ascertain the nature and extent of any real risks, not to attempt to discredit critics or to mount a public relations campaign to improve the company's image. A review of company products or practices that were ultimately found to be harmful in different industries—such as the exposure of employees to harmful chemicals, the polluting of rivers, the tolerance of racial discrimination in the workplace, and the mass promotion of tobacco—shows that concerns were often first raised by a small number of professionals or by a small number of employees or by a small number of activist citizens. Critics do not always have a full and accurate picture, of course, but listening to critics in an effort to learn more about risks to stakeholders is a significant component of corporate responsibility.

When it is not possible to meet all stakeholder needs and legitimate concerns, the very first priority is to avoid doing any serious harm to any of the stakeholders.

Serious harm includes the violation of any basic rights as well as the exposure to any risks which, if understood, would be clearly unacceptable to relevant stakeholders. Some actions or practices are ethically intolerable. The benefits provided to some stakeholders do not justify exposing others to these harms. The benefits to shareholders and to consumers do not justify, for example, the existence of sweatshop conditions for employees in the apparel industry. The basic demand that society makes upon any business is that, in its pursuit of financial interests, it must avoid doing serious harm. This comes first—the highest priority and the first thing to be done in meeting a minimum standard of business ethics.

The priority of avoiding serious harm is the reason why so much of the effort to understand and delineate the ethical responsibilities of businesses is, and needs to be, focused on trying to identify and reduce risks associated with specific business practices. This focus does not deny the obvious benefits provided by business. It is sometimes argued that the ethical commitment should be to a balance between benefit and harm, not to the priority of avoiding harm. The benefit, however, is usually to some stakeholders and the harm to other stakeholders. Consumers and shareholders might benefit, for example, from the release of toxic waste into the environment. It would make more sense to focus on the balance of benefit and harm if the very same people and only the very same people were experiencing both the benefits and the harms. If they then choose to accept the risks of harm, these risks would not be "patently unacceptable."

All risks of harm arising from activities of the company need to be taken seriously.

Other risks of harm to stakeholders not as serious as those that need to be avoided altogether might also result from corporate activities. These, too, should be avoided if possible. Where they cannot be avoided entirely, they should be minimized. Where they cannot be avoided, those who are negatively affected should be appropriately compensated (Principle 5). While the very highest priority is to avoid having serious harm result from company practices or activities, it is important to address any risk of harm. The fact that some risks are not as totally unacceptable as the violations of human rights and the other risks referred to in Principle 6 does not mean that they can legitimately be ignored.

In seeking to achieve a fair distribution of the benefits and burdens of company activities among stakeholders, it is essential to consider the different contributions and vulnerabilities of various stakeholders.

After the application of the "avoiding harm" priority, the next step in stakeholder management is to determine how best to allocate benefits and burdens. The Clarkson Principles recognize "contributions and vulnerabilities" as considerations to be taken into account. A for-profit business can, therefore, appropriately put an emphasis on those who provide the capital to make the business successful. As noted in the introduction to the Clarkson Principles, "there is no reason to think that the conscientious and continuing practice of stakeholder management will conflict with conventional financial performance goals."[5] Stockholders make a major contribution and are vulnerable to loss of their investments. Their comparative standing among stakeholders is high.

Fairness in the distribution of benefits and burdens clearly requires, however, that stockholders not be considered the only stakeholders whose contributions and vulnerabilities are important. Fairness requires that special consideration be given to employees, to those who invest so much of their lives in the company and whose contribution is so central to any success the company achieves. Special consideration must also be given to reducing the burdens on those who are involuntary stakeholders, those affected by company practices even though they did not choose to be associated with the business (for example, community members who might be exposed to toxic chemicals). A fair distribution of benefits and risks also requires that the safety of consumers who are using the company's product be given a very high priority. Stockholders are not the only stakeholders who make a significant contribution or who are vulnerable to being harmed.

THE PHARMACEUTICAL INDUSTRY AND ITS STAKEHOLDERS

Different industries have common stakeholders and common ethical responsibilities. All have employees, for example, and all employees have certain legitimate concerns and interests. When considering responsibilities to employees, therefore, there is often less need to be industry-specific. When, however, the focus is on specific kinds of products and on the marketing of these products, as in this study, it is very important to focus on the key stakeholder groups and the ways in which these stakeholders are or may be affected by industry practices.

Pharmaceutical companies are in the health business. To be more specific, they are in the business of researching, manufacturing, and marketing medicines. Pfizer puts its statement of purpose at the top of its website homepage: "We dedicate ourselves to humanity's quest for longer, healthier, happier lives through innovation in pharmaceutical, consumer and animal health products"[6] Merck describes itself as "a global research-driven pharmaceutical company" that "discovers, develops, manufactures and markets a broad range of innovative products to improve human and animal health."[7] The trade association, Pharmaceutical Research and Manufacturers of America (PhRMA), "represents the country's leading research-based pharmaceutical and biotechnology companies, which are devoted to inventing medicines that allow patients to live longer, healthier, and more productive lives."[8] Being in the medicine business means a responsibility to meet some important and essential needs of the public. Being in the medicine business means that, in addition to the responsibility that all companies have to avoid harm to stakeholders in and by their business practices, the pharmaceutical industry has a responsibility to provide the public with safe, effective, and affordable medical treatments.

In order to understand its marketing responsibilities, it is essential to emphasize that the pharmaceutical industry manufactures and sells prescription drugs, not some other product. Arnold Relman and Marcia Angell make a very important point when they insist that "prescription drugs are not like ordinary goods, and the market for drugs is not like other markets."[9] Ordinary goods or typical consumer products—for example, clothes, cosmetics, beer, electronics—are usually discretionary purchases in way that medicines are not. Among the significant differences between prescription medicines and typical consumer goods, the following are especially noteworthy:

(1) In the case of prescription drugs, physicians make the decisions about whether the patients should use the product. In the case of a typical consumer product, consumers themselves make the decisions about whether to use the product.

(2) Prescription medicines are used to treat or prevent health problems and patients may be at risk of adverse health consequences if the right medication is not used in the right way. Whether a specific typical consumer good is used or not—and how it is used—often has no health-related consequences.

(3) Prescription drugs are often paid for, in part, from shared and limited resources (insurance). Individuals usually pay for typical consumer items from personal or family funds.

(4) Many physicians make decisions about which prescription drugs to use without an awareness of actual costs or how the cost of one medication compares with another. Most consumers of discretionary consumer items make purchases with full knowledge of the cost and often after comparison shopping.

As will be considered more fully later, these kinds of differences have enormous implications regarding the ethical marketing of prescription drugs. Relman and Angell are right on target: "The misconception that drugs and their market are like other goods and markets explains most of the serious problems with the pharmaceutical industry today."[10] Acceptable marketing practices in other industries are not necessarily acceptable practices with regard to prescription drugs. The product is different; the decisions about use are different; the risks are different; the usual method of payment is different.

Pharmaceutical industry stakeholders include all those that are common to any industry—such as stockholders, employees, and contractors. For purposes of understanding the unique role and responsibility of this industry, however, it is important here to focus attention on some stakeholders specific to the pharmaceutical industry. They include the patients who use the medicines; the physicians and other healthcare professionals who prescribe the medicines; the professionals who make determinations related to safety, effectiveness, and appropriate use of the medications (such as clinical researchers, medical journal editors, medical educators); persons with medical needs who do not have access to needed medications; healthcare payers; and healthcare policy makers. The most important questions to be asked about industry marketing practices are questions about the impact on the quality and cost of medical care and on the integrity of medical professionals.

WHAT FOLLOWS

Since prescription drugs are most heavily marketed to medical professionals and to the public, these are the two stakeholder groups to be considered most fully here: medical professionals in their clinical, scientific, and educational roles, and the public both as individual patients and as citizens. The following chapters are devoted to exploring the ethical responsibilities of the pharmaceutical industry in marketing prescription drugs to these two stakeholder groups. The analysis is designed to help clarify what is owed to these key stakeholders, in terms of general responsibilities and in consideration of some specific practices. The risks of harm and the need to provide good medicine both imply definite limits to commercial interests in the marketing of prescription medications.

PART TWO

MARKETING TO HEALTHCARE PROFESSIONALS

3

Drug Companies and Healthcare

Professionals: The Ethics Agenda

My experience was probably similar to that of many others. I went
with a patient to a doctor's appointment a couple of years ago. As
we sat, I began to pay careful attention to what was taking place in
the waiting room. Centered in the room was a television featuring
a series of short educational programs on health-related topics.
The programs were interspersed with commercials, primarily for
prescription drugs. My estimate was that, given the normal waiting time that day, patients on average were exposed to about 10
ads for prescription drugs, without their choice.

In the time that we waited, three sales representatives, from
three different pharmaceutical companies, entered, approached
the receptionist, and handed over their business cards as well as
several small items that might have been pens. One told the receptionist that he had a "last minute" dinner invitation for the doctor.
The other two were carrying bags and took seats in the waiting
room. I suspected that they were waiting for the opportunity to
meet with the doctor while he took a lunch break, and I guessed

that their bags contained copies of studies and other promotional material as well, perhaps, as some samples of medications. I was not in the waiting room long enough to see whether either of the reps was invited in to meet with the doctor.

I had two different impressions of what was going on. One impression, reflected in the practice of the sales representatives seeking the doctor's attention (and using the gifts and invitations to help get it) was of the industry playing up to physicians, where the real power in medicine lies, almost begging for an opportunity to show their wares. The other impression was quite different. The pervasive presence of the pharmaceutical industry that morning, reflected in the waiting room TV's direct-to-consumer advertising of prescription drugs and in the presence of three sales representatives at the same time, gave the impression of the doctor's office as an extension of the industry, an extension of the business of selling drugs. An observer might easily conclude that the industry is clearly in the driver's seat and physicians, knowingly or not, are simply part of the process of selling the company's products.

The relationships that have come to exist between prescribing physicians[2] and the companies that manufacture and market medications inevitably affect the nature and quality of the healthcare provided. The nature of that relationship and its impact on healthcare have recently begun to get much more attention. Now, more than ever before, attention is being paid to the risks these interactions pose to the scientific and ethical integrity of physicians and to their ability to act objectively in their patients' interest. The occasional article of 15–20 years ago has grown to fairly frequent studies and commentaries today.[3]

Much of the early scrutiny was focused on the issue of gift-giving, especially the ways in which the pharmaceutical companies sometimes "wine and dine" physicians in their efforts to get them to listen to their marketing messages. Questions about the appropriateness of physicians accepting such gifts—expense-paid trips, dinners in expensive restaurants, tickets to entertainment, free lunches, items for personal or professional/office use, and samples of medications—have led to efforts for clarifying ethical standards for the medical profession. The American College of Physicians published a position paper on "Physicians and the Pharmaceutical Industry" in 1990[4] and the Council on Ethical and Judicial Affairs of the American Medical Association (AMA), in 1992, published its guidelines on "Gifts to Physicians from Industry." The introductory paragraph of the AMA document included the statement that "Some gifts that reflect customary practices of industry may not be consistent with the Principles of Medical Ethics."[5] The guidelines were designed to help physicians recognize the kinds of gifts that are appropriate and those that are inappropriate to accept.

The ethical guidelines from the early 1990s, however, clearly did not have the effect of reducing or limiting the extent of commercial influence on medicine. Since these guidelines were published, "evidence of industry's influence on medical practice, research, and education has continued to emerge, and physician-industry relationships have multiplied."[6]

Some healthcare professionals have decided that no gifts of any sort should be accepted from the pharmaceutical industry. The "No Free Lunch" movement encourages healthcare providers to recognize and avoid the risks associated with participating in industry promotional activities. "We . . . believe that pharmaceutical promotion should not guide clinical practice, and that over-zealous promotional practices can lead to bad patient care. It is our goal to encourage health care practitioners to provide high quality care based on unbiased evidence rather than on biased pharmaceutical promotion."[7] No Free Lunch encourages physicians to pledge their commitment to say "no" to industry sales representatives, their gifts, and their marketing materials.

The No Free Lunch Pledge reads:

> I, _____, am committed to practicing medicine in the best interest of my patients and on the basis of the best available evidence, rather than on the basis of advertising or promotion.
>
> I therefore pledge to accept no money, gifts, or hospitality from the pharmaceutical industry; to seek unbiased sources of information and not rely on information disseminated by drug companies; and to avoid conflicts of interest in my practice, teaching, and/or research.[8]

DEMANDS FOR CHANGE

The voices of the critics of industry-practitioner relationships are getting stronger and louder. Demands for change are increasingly common. Practices that were rarely discussed previously are now being challenged in ever-widening circles, both among medical professionals and in public. Nevertheless, it is not clear how high a priority is being placed on practical reform in the relationships between drug companies and doctors. While physicians, as individuals and in their associations, may no longer be able to ignore the issues related to their relationships to the drug industry, and while drug companies are being questioned about their marketing practices much more than previously, the changes in behavior, to date, appear to be minimal.

The pharmaceutical industry continues to place a strong emphasis on marketing directly to those who prescribe the medications. In fact, in recent years the number of sales representatives employed by the pharmaceutical companies to promote their products to physicians in the United States has increased significantly, up to about 90,000 full time employees in 2001, one for every 4.7 office-based physicians. The industry invests an estimated $12–$15 billion in marketing to physicians in the United States, over $8,000 for each practicing doctor.[9]

There is significant evidence to show that these promotional activities directed toward physicians by drug companies do, in fact, have a definite impact on the prescribing behavior of physicians.[10] This is not surprising to the lay public, most of whom believe that drug companies would not engage in this activity if it weren't effective, but many physicians continue to insist that their medical judgments and prescribing behavior are not affected by promotional activity[11] and they continue to make use of industry-provided or industry-sponsored education about medications.[12]

Changes in practice may be minor, but changes are occurring in the way the issues are understood and articulated. This constitutes a significant development in clarifying the ethics agenda. While much of the earlier attention was focused on gifts, dinners, and travel, the whole range of interactions between the industry and physicians is now being questioned. Emphasis is now being placed, for example, on the financial relationships that often exist between physicians and industry. Professional judgments, it is noted, are at risk of bias when physicians have financial ties with industry "as researchers, speakers, consultants, investors, owners, partners, employees, or otherwise."[13]

Perhaps the most significant development is that the demand for high ethical standards is being directed toward the industry as well as toward physicians. It is no longer just the question of how healthcare professionals can and should maintain their integrity in the face of industry efforts to sell their products. It is no longer just an emphasis on the professional ethics of physicians. Much more emphasis is now being placed on the ethical standards of the industry, especially in marketing their products to physicians. PhRMA, the trade organization of the brand name pharmaceutical industry, published its voluntary "Code on Interactions with Healthcare Professionals" in 2002.[14] The interest in the industry to protect against inappropriate practices, especially the use of incentives provided to physicians, has been reinforced by the federal Office of Inspector General, which, in an effort to implement anti-kickback statutes more vigorously, published its "OIG Compliance Program Guidance for Pharmaceutical Manufacturers" in 2003.[15] Both industry and physicians are increasingly recognizing that, in the words of David Blumenthal, "in certain respects, the relationships between drug companies and doctors have become embarrassing to both parties and need to change."[16]

Much is being talked about, but not much has yet changed. Marketing medications to physicians is now part of the ethics agenda, but the visits of sales representatives to physician offices continue unabated and the financial connections of physicians with drug companies have probably never been more extensive. It may be that the most obviously inappropriate types of incentives (giving kickbacks to physicians for using company products or providing them with expensive personal gifts and trips) are no longer defended when they occur; many other practices, however, remain a routine part of accepted practice, even though they have been identified as potentially compromising to medical objectivity. Both the PhRMA Code and the AMA guidelines permit many of these interactions to continue and one cannot help but wonder about the seriousness of reform efforts when the AMA's project of educating physicians about the ethics of accepting gifts from industry has been funded, in large part, by the pharmaceutical industry itself![17]

The agenda now is to move the ethics efforts forward:

(1) to examine seriously the issues raised by the various relationships between the pharmaceutical industry and physicians;

(2) to clarify, in general, the nature of companies' ethical responsibilities when marketing medications to physicians;

(3) to assess the available codes and guidelines to determine whether they are adequate to the task of protecting physician objectivity;

(4) to begin to specify what the public, physicians included, should demand of pharmaceutical companies, beyond what is legally required at present;

(5) to move, in general, from being embarrassed about some practices to identifying and implementing good ethics in all the interactions.

PRACTICES NEEDING ATTENTION

There are a variety of practices that the drug industry uses in its interactions with physicians that have been identified as questionable or potentially questionable, actions that need to be submitted to careful ethical analysis and judgment. The concerns that are identified here relate to the nature of the practices and the consequences or impact of these practices; there is little or no attempt to ascertain or critique the motives or intentions behind the actions. Practices can have undesirable consequences even when the intentions are admirable. The following are examples that raise significant ethical questions.

1. Using sales representatives to provide physicians with information about the benefits and risks of the company's drugs

Sales representatives are hired to sell products, while scientific education is designed to be objective and unbiased. There is an inherent threat to scientific objectivity involved in the practice of using sales staff to provide scientific information. Companies, of course, have an incentive to be honest with physicians so that they can keep their good will. On the other hand, there is enormous potential for selectivity in the studies presented. Bias is not the same as explicit deception, but both can lead to a distorted understanding of a drug and its effects. Because so much of the distribution of information about medications is tied to commercial interests, claims like this one from John Abramson need to be taken seriously: "The truth is that American medical practice today is based on scientific evidence as long as the evidence supports commercial interests; but all too often when the science conflicts with commercial interests, science gets nudged aside."[18] Understanding the kind of information pharmaceutical companies owe to physicians is one key to understanding high ethical standards for marketing interactions.

2. Providing gifts to physicians and staff

When sales representatives provide gifts to physicians and their staffs, the concern is how the practice affects the prescribing decisions of physicians and how it might, thereby, affect the quality and cost of healthcare. The gifts are pervasive. The thousands of sales reps who visit physicians rarely, if ever, arrive without bearing some gift or invitation. This issue is the one that has received the most attention to date and continues to require on-going scrutiny. One response has been to distinguish between gifts that benefit patients and gifts that are for the personal benefit of the physician/staff. It needs to be determined whether this distinction does, on careful analysis, address the real issue adequately.

3. Providing free samples of medications

A major component of pharmaceutical marketing to physicians is the distribution of sample medications that physicians can dispense. Many physicians and many patients like the fact that samples are available that can be dispensed free to patients—one reason, perhaps, why this practice has not received the same kind of concentrated attention as other types of "freebies." The practice appears to have a significant impact on decisions to use a particular drug. Because it is available and "free," a drug might be prescribed that would not have been selected if an independent and objective assessment had been made of the drug's effectiveness, risks, cost, and appropriateness, compared with other possible medical treatments. The practice of providing samples requires much more ethical attention than it has received to date.

4. Employing physicians as consultants
5. Employing physicians as speakers in industry-sponsored "educational" programs

Pharmaceutical companies commonly employ physicians (especially those judged to be "opinion leaders") as consultants and/or as speakers to assist them in developing, testing, and marketing their products. These practices, by connecting the physicians to the company's goals through financial and other ties, raise questions about the scientific objectivity of the speakers/consultants themselves in their own practices and in the influence they may have on others. Medical journal editors who seek independent experts to write review articles (articles that summarize a field of study, for example, on the diagnosis and treatment of a particular disease) often have a difficult time finding someone who does not have a consultant and/or speaker relationship with one or more drug companies. Many members of expert panels appointed to write clinical practice guidelines on the treatment of a particular condition have similar relationships.[19] Though physician consultants consistently claim that their scientific judgments are not influenced by their relationships to drug companies, there is good reason to be skeptical of these claims. The need of practicing physicians for unbiased information means that the industry practice of hiring physician opinion leaders as consultants and speakers should be placed high on the ethics agenda.

6. Marketing most aggressively the most profitable medications

Probably few are surprised that, in marketing to physicians, pharmaceutical companies commonly emphasize the product that the company is most interested in selling. The products highlighted, often new ones that still have patent protection, tend to be the more profitable products. They may not always be the most effective ones and, especially if they are new medications, under-standing of their risks of harm is still evolving. It is not surprising that this practice exists, given the sales- and profit-driven nature of marketing. The pharmaceutical industry is a particular kind of business, however, and the full ethical implications for market-ing as part of the medicine business need to be explored much further.

7. Acquiring and using information about the prescribing prac-tice of the individual physician
8. Using sales-based incentives to compensate drug company sales representatives

Through the purchase of pharmacy records, companies are of-ten able to track which physicians prescribe which medications for their patients.[20] This information can then be used to personalize the marketing strategy in meeting with physicians (focusing atten-tion on one particular medical condition, for example, in an effort to get the physicians to switch from one medication to another) and adds an element of sales pressure that might not be there oth-erwise. It is not clear that the professional prescribing decisions of individual physicians should be acquired by companies who use this information to promote their commercial interests. This is another example of a marketing practice that might be more ap-propriate in another industry than in prescription drugs.

Pharmacy record information can also be used to determine how successful the sales representative is in promoting the com-pany's products. On the basis of this information, the company can determine whether, and by how much, prescribing of the company's medications increases after the rep has promoted this product to this physician. The information can also be used, of course, to compute the sales rep's compensation or bonus.

The kind of compensation or reward system that a company uses communicates to employees in a very forceful manner what the company considers important. Pharmaceutical sales represent-atives are typically paid, in part, by commission and/or by bonuses for achieving sales goals. "[B]onuses alone, based on the prescrib-ing patterns of the physicians they cover, can add $30,000 to $50,000 per year to a generous base salary, as long as one moves enough product."[21] Even with the existence of codes of appropriate practices, the company that pays this way may be communicating to sales reps (whether intentionally or not) that achieving the bottom line in sales is much more important than how it gets done.

9. Providing funding for the development of treatment guidelines

Many professional organizations develop clinical guidelines to assist practicing physicians in their treatment of patients with specific medical conditions. Financial support for the development of these guidelines sometimes comes from companies that have a financial interest in the recommendations of the panels. While this practice may not appear at first to be directly related to the marketing of prescription drugs, it is another way companies might have an impact on prescribing decisions. The question of the appropriate role of pharmaceutical companies in the development of treatment guidelines is one of the many conflict-of-interest-related issues that need thorough ethical scrutiny.

10. Providing funding for continuing medical education

Physicians are required to participate in on-going education and much of the budget for continuing medical education is provided by pharmaceutical companies. This long-established practice carries with it the potential for undue influence on the content of educational programs, perhaps even when educational support is provided without any restrictions. Are there any safe ways ("safe" in the sense of protecting against bias in education) in which companies that market to physicians can provide financial support for scientific education?

11. Paying fees to physicians for enrolling their patients in clinical research studies

In their efforts to secure patients as subjects in clinical studies of their drugs, companies have been providing a significant incentive to private physicians (up to several thousand dollars per patient enrolled in some studies) to sign up their patients as subjects.[22] This incentive raises questions and concerns—whether physicians, given the financial self-interest, might be inappropriately influenced in the selection of patients as candidates for the study and whether they might subtly misrepresent the nature of the study and its implications for the patient. It might also make it more difficult for a patient/subject to dis-enroll from a study. As more of the clinical research has moved from academic medical centers to community-based settings and as the number of private practice physicians engaged in finding subjects continues to increase, it is essential to have clear ethical guidance on all research-related interactions between industry and doctors, including this practice of paying fees for enrolling patients. While this might be considered more an issue in research ethics than in marketing ethics, it is another method of establishing financial ties between the companies and healthcare professionals.

This incomplete list of marketing-related practices provides an indication of the range of issues and concerns raised about industry-physician relationships. Only some of these practices will be discussed in more detail in the following chapters, but the discussion is designed to identify the concepts, guiding principles, and methods of analysis that might be used to address other practices as well.

WHAT IS AT STAKE

The list of practices that raise questions about ethical standards is not meant to suggest that there are no benefits at all that result from the marketing relationships of pharmaceutical companies to physicians. Physicians do sometimes gain unbiased and useful information about drugs through marketing-related practices, information which benefits their patients. The question, however, is whether there are unnecessary risks of harm associated with any of these practices and, if so, whether some steps can be taken to reduce these risks. As emphasized earlier, the need to avoid harm should be a high ethical priority for any business. Companies in the medicine business have a responsibility not simply to avoid harm but also to protect and promote high-quality care. The public can legitimately demand that, in marketing their medications, pharmaceutical companies ascertain the likely consequences of various practices and engage only in those practices that are fully compatible with good patient care and with professionalism in the delivery of care.

It is common, when concerns are expressed about any company's marketing methods, for someone else to point out that consumers have to take personal responsibility for their own decisions and actions, that they should not blame the company for their own purchase decisions. This response, whatever its merit in regard to the purchase of consumer items, is not particularly relevant here. Not only are we considering medications (different from consumer items in their potential impact and in the fact that they are more difficult for patients to recognize their benefits and risks on their own), but also the marketing is being done to physicians, who then decide whether to use the medications for patients. Both physicians and consumers need to act responsibly in regard to use and purchase of drugs, of course, but that does not deny or reduce the importance of focusing on the marketing practices of the companies trying to sell the products.

In considering what is at stake in regard to the practices listed above, and in trying to ascertain what might be the best ethical practices, it may be useful to review the major underlying concerns. There are different types of (potential) consequences that need to be kept in mind.

1. Impact on professional and scientific integrity

When companies market medications to physicians, two different worlds meet. The professional responsibility of physicians is defined by their scientific training and by their service commitment to their patients. They are expected to be committed to seeking unbiased information on medications and to putting their patients' well-being above their own self-interest or convenience. The world of marketing, on the other hand, is dominated by the techniques of selling. Products are expected to be presented in the best light possible (without engaging in outright deception) and information that may persuade someone not to use the product need not be included. Selling techniques also include, at times, incentives for the buyer to consider and/or to purchase the product.

Marketing medicines for physicians to prescribe for patients, however, is not the same as marketing consumer products to the public. Pharmaceutical companies need to recognize and respect the nature of medical professionalism. Any of the marketing practices that do not protect and re-enforce medical professionalism have no legitimate place in marketing medicines to doctors. It is primarily this commitment to protecting professional integrity that has led to many of the concerns that have been expressed in recent years about company practices. When professionalism is compromised because of the selling techniques used, harm is done both to the profession and to patients. Physicians have a responsibility to protect themselves from being compromised, and the companies selling medical products have a responsibility to respect and protect professionalism.

2. Impact on the quality of healthcare

The Institute of Medicine has described quality concerns in healthcare as including underuse (failure to provide proven effective medicine), overuse (unnecessary interventions or treatment not indicated by symptoms), and misuse (interventions causing preventable complications).[23] Primary responsibility to prescribe appropriate medications, to avoid the harm done through underuse, overuse, and misuse, rests with individual physicians. Others who influence their prescribing practices have responsibility as well—such as researchers, medical educators, professional organizations and clinical guideline writers, medical journal editors and authors, and insurance companies and pharmacy benefits managers. So also do the companies that market medications.

Evidence-based medicine requires access to the best information available, not just to the information that fits the company's sales goals. Evidence-based medicine also requires freedom from inappropriate influences in the interpretation and application of that information. Because of the inherent connection between professional/scientific integrity and healthcare quality, it is essential that the public, as well as healthcare professionals, pay careful attention to the methods used to market medications to physicians.

3. Impact on the cost of healthcare

The actual financial resources available for healthcare are limited. There are limits to how much employers, government, and individuals are willing to spend. The fact of limited available resources means, in a very real sense, that money spent for one use or one person is not available elsewhere.[24] This is especially true when considering shared resources (private or governmental insurance programs). Because it means that other needs may not be met, spending more than necessary for medical care is both a major health issue and a major ethical issue.

It is often difficult to know precisely when, especially in the long term, a particular treatment is more expensive than alternative approaches or more expensive than necessary. This difficulty is no reason, however, to deny the importance of cost when seeking to understand the potential impact of the ways pharmaceuticals are marketed to physicians. The organizational self-interest of pharmaceutical companies in selling their most profitable medications needs to be counteracted by a strong recognition that unnecessary costs harm the healthcare system and those served by it.

It is important to emphasize that medical drugs are not just like consumer items. If, influenced by marketing techniques, I buy a computer that does not meet my needs, I am not putting my health at risk or endangering the health of others. If it is more expensive than I need, I am not depriving others of a chance to use a computer. If physicians, influenced by marketing, prescribe medications that do not fit the needs of their patients, they may be doing harm (even if unintentional) and they may be placing an unnecessary burden on limited healthcare resources, thus limiting opportunities of others to receive needed healthcare. And the responsibility for this harm rests, as well, with the companies that influence physician prescribing. Marketing medications needs to be recognized as different from marketing optional consumer items.

SOME RELEVANT ETHICS STANDARDS

The following four general standards might be useful in the process of trying to identify more specifically what companies should do in their interactions with medical professionals.

Protect and promote professional integrity by avoiding actions that may place physicians in conflict-of-interest situations.

Respect the scientific nature of medicine.

These first two are specifically related to the nature of medicine and the responsibilities of medical professionals and are central to understanding what the industry owes to medical professionals. They are discussed in the next chapter.

Have a reward system that promotes high ethical standards among sales representatives.

There is much truth to the adage that "ethics is caught rather than taught." What management does is much more important than what management says in communicating to employees the ethical standards of the organization. Employees can usually be expected to adhere to the ethical standards (however high or low) that are consistently demonstrated, consciously or unconsciously, as "the way things are done around here."

Codes of ethics for employees can be an important way of providing clear guidance in regard to expected behavior. But, by itself, a code is not likely to be effective. It needs to be consistent with, and reinforced by, all the other messages sent by management to employees, especially by company policies and practices. Employees tend to learn very quickly what kind of behavior is encouraged and rewarded. The rewards can be anything from financial rewards, such as a compensation increase or promotion to a new position, to verbal commendations. When, for example, someone who consistently plays down the risks associated with the use of the company's medications is rewarded because he or she achieves sales goals, the company is telling the sales staff that sales numbers, not objectivity in presentation, is what is desired (even if sales representatives are "taught" the importance of providing accurate information on risks).

The public should demand that pharmaceutical companies assess their reward practices for sales representatives to ensure that they are truly rewarding the kind of behavior, and only the kind of behavior, that is compatible with the scientific and service nature of medical practice.

Seek outside assistance in working out the practical ethical implications of the general standards.

In 2002, Premier, Inc., a group purchasing organization which provides purchasing and other functions to hospitals and healthcare systems, hired Kirk Hanson, a business ethicist, to develop a report on good ethical practices for the group purchasing industry. It was agreed from the beginning that Hanson would have access to any documents and individuals within Premier that he wished, that he would have complete independence in developing his recommendations, and that the report would be made public upon completion. When the Board accepted the report, they made it public and directed management to begin to implement the recommendations.[25]

Premier's practice in this case recognized that, at least at times, it is important to get outside assistance in identifying the best ethical practices for an industry or a company. It is often very difficult for those on the inside, who are used to established ways of doing things, to recognize all of the issues related to their practices. And we all tend to be biased judges in our own cases. Pharmaceutical companies that are interested in identifying the best ethical practices would do well to seek outside and independent assistance. Given the self-interest of the industry to maintain practices that have long been part of a very profitable business, ethical objectivity seems to require that specific practices be evaluated by outsiders.

Physicians have a conflict of interest when their interests or commitments compromise their independent judgment or their loyalty to patients.[1]

4

Medical Professionalism and
Scientific Integrity

In an essay in *The New York Times,* Abigail Zuger provided an example of a physician's prescribing behavior being influenced by exposure to pharmaceutical marketing. She tells the story of a physician friend. He is someone who deplores the extent to which such marketing has affected the prescribing habits of colleagues but sees himself as a man of science, independence, and integrity who will not be swayed by the potential bias of marketing. He takes advantage of everything the companies offer—the small gifts, the dinners, "the occasional all-expense-paid jaunt to a balmy resort to participate in a focus group."[2] He participates in company-sponsored educational programs.

When a particular new HIV drug came out some time ago, this physician was initially skeptical of its value but took advantage of the various opportunities that the company presented to learn about the drug. As time passed and more studies were done, the evidence suggested that the new drug was not really effective and medical advisory groups began to recommend that it not be used. Zuger concludes the story this way:

My friend, nothing if not conscientious, went through his list of patients to identify those with HIV infection who were on the drug, so that he could contact them and change their pills. The next time I ran into him he was a little subdued, newly conscious of the power of subliminal advertising. "It turns out I had an awful lot of people on that silly drug," he said. "I honestly can't imagine how that happened."[3]

As publicly traded for-profit businesses, pharmaceutical companies must focus on providing return to investors, but this needs to be balanced by other responsibilities to other stakeholders. As manufacturers and marketers of medicines, their key stakeholders include the medical professionals to whom they market their drugs and with whom they work in testing drugs. In this chapter, I explore some aspects of what it means, in a general ethical framework, to respect the professional and scientific integrity of medical practitioners, researchers, and educators and to avoid any actions that might tend to compromise or undermine their integrity.

CONFLICT-OF-INTEREST SITUATIONS

In considering the possible negative consequences of the ways in which pharmaceutical companies interact with physicians, the most important concept to highlight is "conflict of interest." Conflict-of-interest analysis is commonly used to help clarify responsibilities in business, public service, and the professions. It underlies standards and policies on the acceptance of gifts and honoraria, on relationships to contractors or suppliers, and on the use of personal incentives to influence behavior.

A conflict-of-interest situation exists whenever someone has a relationship or is otherwise subject to influences that have a significant potential to lead that person to act contrary to his or her professional or ethical responsibility. Other interests are present that are or may be antagonistic to professional and/or ethical responsibilities and these other interests are substantial enough that they reasonably might affect her/his judgments or actions.[4] While there is often an emphasis on financial matters in conflict-of-interest analysis, there are a variety of other factors that might also influence persons to act contrary to their primary responsibilities. The opposing interest can even be one that does not directly benefit the individuals personally but contributes to something that is of importance to them.

According to Marc Rodwin, "Physicians have a conflict of interest when their interests or commitments compromise their independent judgment or their loyalty to patients."[5] They fail to live up to their professional responsibility when self-interest or similar influences bias their judgment or otherwise compromise their service to their patients. Since professionals do not ordinarily deliberately choose to put other interests above their responsibilities, it is important to focus on the situations in which this might happen unconsciously, the kinds of settings in which professional standards might well become compromised despite the best of intentions. As regards the ethics of marketing drugs, the issue is not "overt corruption such as fraud, bribes, office-buying, or kickback. Yet what we are concerned about is equally problematic, far subtler, and largely hidden from sight."[6] Physicians' conflicts of interest contribute to bias; they compromise professionalism; they breed distrust.

Some examples of conflict-of-interest situations outside of the marketing of drugs include

(1) A purchasing department employee is given tickets to a major sports event from a vendor who does business with the employee's organization.

(2) The brother of a city council member is the owner of a development company that is seeking a city contract.

(3) The department manager is romantically involved with a person s/he supervises (and whose work performance s/he evaluates).

(4) The speaker at an education program on the uses of genetic research is selected and paid for by a company that markets genetic tests.

(5) The CEO of the hospital buying group (which negotiates contracts for products for many hospitals) owns stock in a product supplier with whom the buying group does business.

(6) A member of the Institutional Review Board (the committee that reviews proposed research to protect the rights

of human subjects) has done joint research previously
with the principal investigator of the research project
under review.
(7) The chair of the hospital Ethics Case Consultation Team
is a good friend and golfing companion of the physician
who requests a consultation.

In each of these cases, there is a risk that objectivity will be compromised—because of the situation, not necessarily because of the
lack of commitment to objectivity on the part of those involved.
In all of these cases, there is a risk that the individuals involved will
fail to carry out their primary responsibilities. The risk of bias and
of compromise would be much less if the conflicting interest were
not present. In most instances, allowing oneself to be influenced
inappropriately is neither recognized nor intentional; one does
not deliberately choose to go against the primary responsibility.
Rather, the nature of the context inclines one to other interests,
often without conscious awareness.

Since most professionals do not deliberately choose to act
against their primary responsibility, the solution is not simply to
emphasize the importance of good character or right intention
or pure motives. It is more important to address the conflict-of-
interest situation than to rely upon personal ethical integrity or
strength of character alone to prevent questionable decisions or
actions as a result of conflicting interests. It is the context or situation that inclines one to other interests and the solution is to avoid
or control the context or situation. In the story at the beginning
of the chapter, the physician was surprised that he had prescribed
the particular medication as often as he had. His commitment
to what is best for his patients appeared to be very strong, but it
did not prevent other influences from affecting his prescribing
behavior. He was not aware until later just how much effect the
marketing strategy had had on him.

It is sometimes said that conflict-of-interest situations cannot
be totally avoided. There may be some truth in this statement, but
this element of truth does not justify a reduced commitment to
identifying and avoiding conflict-of-interest situations whenever
possible. For individuals or groups to maintain their professional

integrity and to act in accord with high ethical standards, they must take conflict-of-interest situations very seriously. They need to avoid or eliminate these situations, if possible, and minimize or control the impact of the opposing interest, if the situations cannot be avoided. The starting point is to recognize these situations, whatever form they take and whenever they exist. Unless they are recognized, they will neither be avoided nor managed.

Many of the ways in which pharmaceutical companies market their products to physicians appear to involve physicians in conflict-of-interest situations. Having free samples of medications on hand may influence their judgment about which medication should be "tried" first. Being employed as a consultant to or as a speaker for a particular company may incline one to be partial to that company's products. Getting information about a new drug's effectiveness and risks through company-sponsored information may affect the physician's objectivity (with or without the acceptance of personal gifts). If a friendly on-going relationship is established with a company's sales representative, the physician may favor that company's drugs without conscious awareness.

It is not unusual for physicians to insist that their professional judgment is, in fact, not influenced by gifts from and by other interactions with pharmaceutical companies. This belief continues even when studies show that physician behavior is clearly influenced by these relationships. "Despite the confidence of physicians in their ability to resist efforts by drug companies to affect their behavior . . . a substantial body of theoretical and empirical literature . . . suggests that many physicians are mistaken."[7] There are different explanations for this continuing belief. One is that "humans are vulnerable to a powerful, unconscious 'self-serving bias.'"[8] We do not always see ourselves as we really are. Professionals, trained to think in terms of their professional responsibility, can exaggerate the extent to which they are unaffected or unlikely to be affected by other considerations. A second possible explanation is confusion regarding the nature of influence, seeing it in terms of intention more than in terms of results. Because they do not intend that their behavior will be influenced by the interactions with pharmaceutical companies, physicians might conclude that their actions are, in fact, not so influenced.

It is quite common in business codes of ethics to consider the value of a gift or the extent of a financial interest when determining what is to be avoided. Corporate policies on accepting gifts from suppliers, for example, often distinguish between gifts of nominal value (such as an inexpensive pen with the company's logo), which may be accepted, and gifts of greater value, which may not be accepted. Disclosure policies in research settings sometimes require that investigators report "significant financial interests" in the company sponsoring the study. The distinction between nominal and significant value makes some obvious sense. Not all interests that are potentially antagonistic to professional or ethical responsibilities should be considered the same. Some, it is argued, are too insubstantial and/or too remote to be reasonably expected to affect judgment or behavior.

On the other hand, it may be that the monetary value of competing interest is not relevant. Some have argued that gifts, regardless of their value, can produce a sense of indebtedness that may affect behavior: "When a gift or gesture of any size is bestowed, it imposes on the recipient a sense of indebtedness. The obligation to directly reciprocate, whether or not the recipient is conscious of it, tends to influence behavior. . . . Feelings of obligation are not related to the size of the initial gift or favor."[9]

It is important to emphasize that the concern is not that physicians will deliberately choose to prescribe something that they know is not appropriate for their patients because of gifts or other relationships with drug companies. The concern is, rather, that these interactions and relationships will influence medical judgment in subtle and unrecognized ways, and that they will lead to prescribing medications that are not the most appropriate for patients. The primary responsibility for attending to conflicts of interest rests with the medical profession itself (individual physicians, professional associations, medical educators, etc.). Because conflicts of interest always threaten professionalism and the quality of care, healthcare professionals have a responsibility to avoid conflict-of-interest situations, if possible. And they have a responsibility to reduce the likelihood that they will act contrary to their professional responsibility when, for some reason, conflict-of-interest situations cannot be avoided.

Others have corresponding ethical obligations. All who interact with healthcare professionals have a serious responsibility to avoid placing these professionals in unnecessary conflict-of-interest situations. The public need not accept the view that businesses may use any personal enticements that do not violate the law in marketing their products to professionals and that it is up to professionals to resist being compromised. Rather, the public should insist that those who market to professionals accept a responsibility to respect the integrity of that profession and relate to it in ways that do not contribute to bias or professional compromise.

Pharmaceutical companies have an ethical responsibility to avoid placing clinicians in unnecessary conflict-of-interest situations because, in part, of the essential need to avoid risks of serious harm to key stakeholders. As noted in the discussion of the Clarkson Principles in chapter 2, companies should avoid altogether activities that "give rise to risks which, if clearly understood, would be patently unacceptable to relevant stakeholders." Risks are not just risks of physical harm. For physicians, the risk of compromising their professional integrity is patently unacceptable. It is a true and serious harm when physicians, even unknowingly, write prescriptions influenced by interests that reduce their ability to be objective in responding to their patients' needs.

There is another consideration that reinforces and strengthens the responsibility of pharmaceutical companies to avoid placing prescription writers in conflict-of-interest situations. Because they are in the medicine business, these companies have a direct responsibility to patients (another key stakeholder group) to contribute to their receiving the right or best medications for their circumstances. Anything that has a reasonable likelihood of undermining the independence and objectivity of physicians to make medication decisions on the basis of the best available scientific evidence is out of place.

It is important to analyze carefully the various ways pharmaceutical companies and their representatives interact with physicians in order to determine whether any of these interactions place physicians in conflict-of-interest situations. If so, the burden of proof is on those who argue that these sorts of interactions should continue. Occasionally, it may be justified to act in ways that contribute to some conflict-of-interest situations because the actions are necessary to achieve some other important or essential goals. In these cases, the company's responsibility is to keep the conflicts as insubstantial as possible and to assist in finding methods of preventing physician behavior that is actually antagonistic to the best interests of patients. Care must always be taken, of course, not to conclude too quickly that something that contributes to a conflict of interest is "necessary." Those who claim that a conflict of interest is necessary carry the burden of proof.

One common way of trying to manage conflict-of-interest situations is to require disclosure of any financial (and other) relationships that have the potential to introduce bias and undermine objectivity. Disclosure is the commonly used method of trying to manage conflicts in medical education and publications in medical journals. The speaker or writer is expected to disclose any financial relationships with companies whose products are being discussed. It is important to remember, however, that disclosure alone does not significantly reduce the risk of bias or other compromise of professional standards. Rather, it simply serves as a warning that the risk exists and that the audience should be aware. Given the great difficulty in detecting in most cases that a presentation is biased, disclosure is not likely to be sufficient by itself to protect the integrity of medicine.

Disclosure is even less of a solution in the doctor's office. If a doctor told the patient that he or she had just gotten some information from a drug company rep (or a company speaker) about a new medication and would like to try it, what should a patient do with this information? Disclosure has limited value only in those situations where both the one doing the disclosing and the one being disclosed to are aware that the fact being revealed might mean biased judgment and are able to evaluate the extent and consequences of bias.

RESPECTING SCIENTIFIC INTEGRITY

"Medicine . . . rests on the promise of utmost objectivity, the closest possible scrutiny of potential confusions or biases. It is thanks to this ethic that we aren't being bled for every ailment under the sun."[10] Scientific medicine requires that physician have access to and make use of unbiased and scientifically valid studies. The general ethical standard is that the individuals and groups engaged in scientific study and in interpreting the results of scientific studies to physicians be scientifically qualified and be dedicated to the pursuit of truth and objectivity.

In an important book on threats to scientific integrity, Sheldon Krimsky, using the earlier work of Robert Merton, identifies the values and norms underlying science as universalism, communalism, disinterestedness, and organized skepticism. For science to function at its best, these values and norms should be accepted and applied as basic ethical commitments.[11] It is relevant here to consider, especially, the meaning of a commitment to the norms of communalism and disinterestedness.

"Communalism" refers to "the common ownership of the fruits of scientific investigation."[12] The findings of science are, normally at least, the results of collaborative work; different researchers contribute to the evolving picture. Science is public in the sense that it needs to be open; it needs to permit different researchers to test and retest theories and applications. Most important, it is a public project in the sense that science involves public service. The benefits should be for the whole community. Scientific findings should be communicated widely and private property rights that restrict this kind of communication in science should be kept to a minimum. Proprietary secrets and other methods of restricting access to scientific information are at odds with the ethos of true science. Medical knowledge and information is and should be treated as "a public good measured by its potential to improve our health" and not "a commodity, measured by its commercial value."[13] The extensive and pervasive relationships between industry and universities in recent years constitute a major threat to this scientific value.

"Disinterestedness" means not being unduly influenced by self-interest. "It requires that scientists apply the methods, perform the analysis, and execute the interpretation of results without considerations of personal gain, ideology, or fidelity to any cause other than the pursuit of truth."[14] Scientists cannot, of course, be totally without personal interests. Disinterestedness means a profound and protected commitment to objectivity, to not permitting personal interests to bias the methods used, the analysis made, and the reporting done. Disinterestedness goes hand-in-hand with communalism. The protection against bias in science is maintained largely by being "a community-driven process."[15]

On the other hand, science driven by commercial interests is wide open to bias. Under the influence of commercial interests, researchers and research organizations are tempted to interpret everything in terms of the potential bottom-line impact. When commercial interests dominate, they affect the research agenda. Since, for example, it is anticipated that there will be more profit in developing cancer medications than in ensuring a healthy environment, "vastly more resources are put into the cellular and genetic basis of cancer than into environmental factors."[16] Commercial interests likewise affect the dissemination of the scientific findings: the drug studies published in even the most prestigious medical journals sometimes contain a scientifically unjustifiable "spin" favorable to corporate interests.[17] Similar to other kinds of conflicts of interest, the loss of disinterestedness among researchers is not normally something that is consciously or deliberately chosen.

The implications of these ethical norms for the science that is done by employees of the pharmaceutical industry are not the primary concern here. Rather, as part of the effort to understand the proper relationship of the industry to medical professionals, I want to direct attention to two different ways in which industry relates to medical professionals. First is the use of science in marketing to physicians. In these marketing efforts, pharmaceutical companies present results of scientific studies in their sales materials. The companies are seeking to sell their products. In a typical approach to marketing, a commitment to providing complete and unbiased information is often subordinated to the interest in selling the product. Selling strategies are not driven by a commitment to objectivity. There can be a major difference, even a conflict, between the commitment to good science (reporting with disinterested openness and objectivity) and the commitment to marketing (emphasizing the information most likely to make the sale). Common marketing strategy does not fit scientific medicine. The public can and should demand that, in all marketing that pharmaceutical companies do to physicians, standards other than the typical marketing ones apply. Specific practices need to be reviewed to ascertain how well they reflect respect for the scientific nature of medicine.

Second, since the marketing of drugs to healthcare professionals makes such extensive use of clinical studies, there is a need to consider the relationships of industry to clinical investigators working in university medical centers or in the community. These researchers, even when doing company-sponsored research, are scientists and physicians whose primary commitment should be to good medicine and good science. Their responsibility to the public good takes priority over any private interests, whether their own or those of the company that is sponsoring the research. As expressed in the Code of Ethics of the American Academy of Pharmaceutical Physicians, physician investigators have a responsibility to "support the dissemination only of scientifically sound information from clinical trials and other investigations, without regard to study outcomes, for the benefit of medicine and science."[18] Companies have a corresponding responsibility to interact with clinical investigators only in those ways that protect and encourage the development and dissemination of scientifically sound information.

Industry needs to respect the integrity of science. In general, this means avoiding any practices or policies that make it more difficult for investigators to serve the public interest and to maintain high standards of objectivity. Similar to physicians in their clinical practice, most medical scientists are convinced that financial interests do not and will not compromise their scientific objectivity or affect their research in other ways. It is not unusual, for example, for investigators to think that owning stock in or having a consulting contract with a company sponsoring their research presents no serious risk to their scientific integrity. As with practicing physicians, this self-perception may be inaccurate.

There appears to be an increasing recognition of the importance of taking conflict-of-interest situations in research very seriously. After a 17-year-old subject in a research project died in 1999 at the University of Pennsylvania, the investigation revealed that both the principal investigator and the university had stock in the company that would profit from the subsequent approval of the treatment being investigated.[19] As a result, many are wondering why such situations are allowed to occur. In 2004, Harvard Medical School approved a new, more stringent policy. Harvard researchers are not permitted "to have a financial interest in a company and conduct clinical research on a technology owned or obligated to that company."[20] Regardless of how clearly investigators themselves recognize them, there are risks to the integrity of science involved in industry-investigator relationships. Both they and the companies that sponsor the research need to take these risks seriously.

Some of the more specific implications of what it means to respect the integrity of medical research will be discussed in later chapters, especially in chapter 9. Two general ethical imperatives are noted here, however, to provide an initial sense of what it means to respect the integrity of science when companies market to physicians and engage outside scientists and physicians in research.

One imperative is that companies not abuse the meaning and purpose of research by masquerading marketing as research. Studies are often done on drugs that already have received FDA approval and are on the market (sometimes called Phase IV studies). Sometimes these studies are done for very legitimate and necessary reasons, but some are designed not so as to gain valid information as to market the drugs. In some Phase IV studies, "sponsors pay doctors to put patients on drugs and answer a few questions about how they fared. There is no randomization and no comparison group, so it is impossible to draw any reliable conclusions."[21] While they have no scientific validity, such "studies" help to achieve the marketing goal of making doctors and patients more familiar with the drug. It is an abuse of science to use human subjects and to involve clinical investigators in projects that have no scientific merit.

A second general imperative is that companies respect the need for science to be open and public. One concern is the practice sometimes employed by industry that requires investigators not publish their findings without the written consent of the company sponsoring the research.[22] This appears to be incompatible with respect for the integrity of the scientific undertakings and at odds with what is owed to medical professionals. Another concern is the reluctance to publish the results of studies when these results are not favorable to the company's product. Good science needs to be both public and disinterested.

The primary statements of the industry's own understanding of its ethical responsibilities in its relationships to medical professionals are two sets of standards published by PhRMA, the industry trade association, in 2002: The "PhRMA Code on Interactions with Healthcare Professionals" and the "PhRMA Principles on Conduct of Clinical Trials and Communication of Clinical Trial Results." The next chapter is a review of the first of these, which addresses issues in marketing-related interactions. The second is considered in chapter 9.

5

They [the PhRMA guidelines] would limit the value of gifts to less than one hundred dollars, and require that the gifts be relevant to patient care—like textbooks. But the guidelines don't ... bother to tell us why drug companies should be giving gifts to doctors in the first place, when the costs will just be added on to drug prices. The guidelines also permit more extravagant gifts and junkets if they can be construed as furthering an educational or research purpose.[1]

The Industry's Code: Not Good Enough

The "PhRMA Code on Interactions with Healthcare Professionals," published in 2002, is a very significant document. It represents an acknowledgment, on the part of the industry, that laws and governmental regulations are not sufficient to provide full guidance to what is good ethical practice. It is a recognition, in effect, that some of the concerns that have been raised about marketing practices need to be addressed. With this Code, the industry has made a public ethics statement, identifying the kinds of activities that it finds acceptable and the kinds of activities that it thinks are not appropriate.

The Code, included at the end of this chapter, merits careful study and reflection. It provides an opportunity to understand the industry's own view of its ethical responsibilities in marketing to healthcare professionals and in related interactions with them. It also provides an opportunity to assess the adequacy of the guidelines, to determine how well they address the concerns that have been raised and whether they represent the approach to marketing that is required by a commitment to good healthcare, good science, and good ethics.

WHAT THE CODE INCLUDES AND DOES NOT INCLUDE

Keeping in mind the range of concerns identified in chapter 3 and the ethical responsibilities to healthcare professionals discussed in chapter 4, it is useful to begin with a few observations on the types of practices that the Code addresses, how it addresses these, and what the Code does not include.

> 1. *The Code does not propose any fundamental changes in the nature, purpose, or frequency of interactions with healthcare professionals. Rather, it delineates between appropriate and inappropriate behaviors within these interactions, primarily by identifying the types of gifts and other inducements that may and may not be offered to healthcare professionals.*

As expressed in the preamble and in section 1, the Code is seen as directly related to the industry's mission of helping patients live longer and healthier lives through the development and marketing of medicines. The purpose of the Code is to clarify the ethical boundaries needed to keep the focus on benefiting patients:

> *This Code is to reinforce our intention that our interactions with healthcare professionals are to benefit patients and to enhance the practice of medicine. The Code is based on the principle that a healthcare professional's care of patients should be based, and should be perceived as being based, solely on each patient's medical needs and the healthcare professional's medical knowledge and experience. (preamble)*

It is not surprising, but it remains worthy of note, that the industry's response to the concerns that have been raised about how marketing to physicians might be affecting medical practice is to repeat its belief that such marketing contributes to better patient care. The approach taken in the Code is much more like the approach taken by the AMA (that there is a need to address some specific questionable practices in the industry's relationships with physicians and other healthcare professionals) than the approach taken by those more critical of the industry (that there is a need to recognize that the very nature of pharmaceutical marketing to professionals threatens professional objectivity and good healthcare). The Code seems, therefore, to be more a defense of the status quo than a reform document.

The Code recognizes that a variety of different non-research interactions—informational presentations sponsored by the company, education provided by others that the company supports financially, the hiring of healthcare professionals as consultants, the training of healthcare professionals to be speakers at company programs, the provision of scholarships for educational programs, and the gifts and social amenities provided to professionals—all relate to the company's marketing efforts. Important ethical issues are addressed in regard to each, but the Code does not call for any reduction in the number or types of interactions.

2. The key method used to establish limits in the practice of providing gifts or other inducements to healthcare professionals is the distinction between items that are primarily for the benefit of patients (which are permitted, unless of substantial value or given more often than on "an occasional basis") and items which are primarily for the personal benefit of the healthcare professional (which are not permitted).

The heavy emphasis put on this distinction is evident when examples are given of the application of the Code in the "Frequently Asked Questions" section that is appended to the Code. Giving stethoscopes or books on patient care to healthcare professionals is compatible with the Code because these items primarily benefit patients (as long as these sorts of items are not of substantial value—over $100—and are only occasionally offered). Items such as golf balls or bookstore gift certificates, on the other hand, should not be offered even if valued under $100, because they primarily benefit the professional, not the patient.

This distinction between patient benefit and the personal benefit of the physician is also found in the standards of the AMA.[2] This distinction is understandable, based as it is on an understanding of the physician as someone who is expected to subordinate his or her personal interests to the professional responsibility to serve the patient. Putting patient benefit before personal benefit is, indeed, a fundamentally important component of medical professionalism. That does not necessarily mean, however, that this distinction is the key to understanding the ethical impact of any gifts or advantages given to physicians by the industry that is seeking to influence their practice. As will be explained later in this chapter, it is ethically questionable and risky to think that the simple fact that gifts may benefit patients prevents physicians from compromising professional judgment or behavior.

Since the Code does recognize that even those gifts that benefit patients and not the physician personally should be of limited value and should not be offered frequently, there may be an implicit recognition that the difference between patient benefit and physician personal benefit is not the only important consideration. Apparently, even gifts that benefit patients can influence physician behavior inappropriately. If this were not the case, there would be no need for limits on value or frequency. Despite this implicit acknowledgement, however, the Code as a whole is based on the belief that the distinction is valid and important.

3. The Code places limits on the kinds of meals that may be provided in conjunction with company-sponsored presentations. Meals may be presented if they are occasional, modest by local standards, in a setting conducive to the informational communication, and if they do not include the guest of the healthcare professional. No entertainment or recreational activities may be offered in conjunction with such programs. (section 2)

A long-standing symbol of questionable practices is the "wining and dining" of physicians (and their guests) at expensive restaurants. Typically, in exchange for the dinner, physicians are expected to listen to a presentation on a company product. The Code limits the value of the "free meal" and emphasizes that the program should be informational rather than entertaining. It addresses the kind of incentives (permitting but limiting the personal benefits to physicians) that can be used to entice physicians to attend company-sponsored programs. Meals are acceptable within limits.

The industry apparently does not see any need to change in any significant ways their efforts to inform physicians through these sorts of programs. It does not address, at least in this Code, the kinds of protections that must be put in place to guarantee scientific accuracy of information or the kinds of disclosures that should be made to attendees. There is nothing that even acknowledges the widely held conviction that there is an inherent conflict when a company markets its products at the same time that is seeks to provide scientifically objective information about these products.

> *4. The Code makes it clear that, when a company provides financial support for educational meetings that are sponsored and organized by others, the organizers, not the company, are to have control over the selection of content, of the faculty, and of the educational materials. Any financial assistance given to support those attending such events should be given to the sponsors, not to individual attendees, and should be used to cover the conference fee rather than the cost of travel or lodging. (sections 3.a and 3.b)*

The Code permits pharmaceutical companies to provide financial support for medical education programs, describing such programs as having the potential to contribute to improvements in patient care. The industry recognizes two concerns that have frequently been expressed about corporate support for medical education: (1) that companies might exert influence in terms of speakers or topics; and (2) that attendance support might lead to a sense of indebtedness among those participants who benefit from this support, a sense of indebtedness that could unknowingly affect prescribing behavior. The Code addresses both of these concerns and does so in a way that, at least at the level of explicit influence, seems adequate. In approving financial support for educational programs provided by others, the Code does not acknowledge any serious risks associated with more subtle influences on healthcare professionals by industry support of professional medical education. I will return to this issue in a later chapter.

LIMITING PHYSICIAN PERSONAL BENEFITS IS NOT ENOUGH

Reflections on conflicts of interest (begun in chapter 4) are the most useful and important ones for clarifying the ethical responsibility of the pharmaceutical industry in marketing medicines to physicians. In general, a conflict of interest exists whenever someone is subject to influences that have a significant potential to lead that person to act contrary to his or her professional or ethical responsibility. The person may be aware of this significant influence or not; the conflict exists in either case. The person may have knowingly placed him- or herself in this situation or may have tried to avoid it; the conflict exists in either case. In one sense, the existence of a conflict of interest does not mean that the individuals in these situations have failed in their responsibility; rather, it means that they are at a higher risk of doing so. In another sense, however, unnecessarily increasing the risk that they or someone else will violate their responsibility is itself a failure to ensure that priorities are kept straight. A commitment to good ethical practices means preventing conflicts of interest whenever possible and, if some are unavoidable, putting mechanisms in place to manage them rigorously. Any industry promoting its products to healthcare professionals has a responsibility to avoid placing these professionals in conflicts of interest, if possible.

The pharmaceutical industry recognizes its responsibility to avoid placing healthcare professionals in conflicts of interest, but its understanding of what this means, as reflected in the Code, is incomplete. It is clear that gifts that are of personal benefit and value to healthcare professionals raise a very significant risk that they will put their own self-interests above the needs of their patients. The industry recognizes that such gifts should be avoided, at least those beyond minimal value. It is not necessarily true, however, that gifts designed to benefit patients (a stethoscope, an anatomical model, or a book on some healthcare issue) are that much safer ethically. In the first place, the distinction does not identify a major difference. What helps the professional in providing patient care also helps that professional personally. If a company provides something physicians can use in patient care, it means that the physicians or their practices do not have to purchase that item. Further, and more important, individuals often feel a sense of gratitude or appreciation when something is provided that they can use, whether it is something of personal benefit or something that assists them in their professional work. Gifts of all sorts establish the identity of the donor in the recipient's mind in a positive way and this feeling toward the giver, even if not a conscious feeling, involves a sense of obligation that can and does affect behavior.[3] Gifts from pharmaceutical companies to physicians, including gifts that can be used for patient benefit, can have a subtle but very real influence on judgment and action.

Good policies on conflict of interest recognize that, generally, the best way of addressing the risks associated with conflicts of interest is by preventing the conflicts from occurring. If that is not possible, those who have such conflicts should not be making important decisions. The need is to mitigate the risk, not to question the intent or motivations behind the behavior that contributes to a conflict. A conflict-of-interest policy is simply about reducing risks of behavior contrary to professional or ethical responsibility. Consider the case of a city council member whose sibling is part owner of a development company that is being considered for a city contract. This council member clearly has a conflict of interest and a good policy requires that he or she abstain from a role in decision making in this case. The integrity of the councilperson or of the family member is not being impugned by the policy that requires that the member abstain and the policy does not suggest that this particular development company cannot submit a good proposal. It is both reasonable and important to have such conflict-of-interest policies because they protect the quality of public service by reducing the likelihood that interests contrary to one's primary responsibility will influence behavior. It is unnecessarily risky to allow a person to exercise (even shared) decision-making authority in a situation where significant influences, contrary to the primary responsibility, might well be at work.

To maintain trust in any organization, it is important to be concerned about anything that may give the appearance of a conflict of interest. The public can have more confidence in the city council if policy prevents a council member from participating in a decision on a contract with a company run by a family member. On the other hand, the lack of such a policy makes it much easier for the public to suspect that council members subordinate the public good to private interests.

In pharmaceutical industry ethics, the issue is not whether the gifts provided to physicians can be used to benefit patients. The issue is not whether the company is sincerely seeking to improve patient care. It is not even whether the specific products that the sales representative is promoting when using such gifts would be judged by qualified independent professionals to be best for treating some specific conditions. Rather, the issue is whether the Code permits practices that are at odds with the industry's commitment to the "principle that a healthcare professional's care of patients should be based, and should be perceived as being based, solely on each patient's medical needs and the healthcare professional's medical knowledge and experience" (statement made in the preamble to the PhRMA Code). This commitment requires that companies not risk the possibility that gifts will affect the independence and objectivity of a prescribing physician.

The distinction in the PhRMA Code between items that serve patient interests and items that are for the personal benefit of the practitioner does not have the great significance that the Code gives it. The public can legitimately expect that those companies truly committed to high-quality patient care will be very careful to avoid all actions that might influence physicians to act on the basis of any factors other than professional responsibility. The industry has recognized that it has a responsibility to avoid placing physicians in conflict-of-interest situations. It now needs to recognize that the application of this ethical principle in the Code is not adequate.

One of the problems associated with allowing the distinction between patient benefit and the personal benefit of the physician to play such a decisive role in the Code is that it radically limits the types of interactions that need to be submitted to conflict-of-interest analysis. Pharmaceutical companies define themselves as being in the business of developing and marketing medications that help patients. They naturally see their marketing efforts, therefore, as falling into the category of patient benefit. It may very well be that it is because the industry has identified the activities related to the personal benefit of physicians as needing the most careful ethical scrutiny that the Code says little or nothing about many of the other issues raised about marketing to physicians. The Code does not address, for example:

- *standards for avoiding bias in the promotional materials used;*
- *the question of marketing off-label uses;*
- *the use of information about a physician's personal prescribing record;*
- *the issue of promoting more expensive medications;*
- *policy on compensating the sales force.*

It is not so much a Code that addresses the major ethical issues raised about marketing medications to healthcare professionals as it is a Code on what kind of benefits and financial support can be provided to healthcare professionals. The latter is needed, but it is only a small part of marketing ethics.

As the first widely promoted industry effort to address ethical issues raised about marketing medications to healthcare professionals, the "PhRMA Code on Interactions with Healthcare Professionals" is a start, but only a start. Though it is a set of voluntary guidelines (that is, not mandated by legal requirements), the approach taken in the Code reflects the concerns found in legal regulations and in prosecutions. Legal concerns have focused on arrangements that might be considered bribes (money or a favor given in order to influence behavior) or kickbacks (returning in money or favors part of the income from what is sold). It appears as though the Code was written from the perspective of the need to avoid the types of gifts and compensation arrangements that might be construed as bribes or kickbacks. This is an understandable approach, but it is not sufficient.

THE NEED FOR MORE ADEQUATE ETHICAL STANDARDS

The PhRMA Code is not sufficient as a statement of the ethical responsibilities involved in marketing drugs to physicians because it is much too narrowly focused in its understanding of ethics and much too limited in the issues addressed. It needs to be expanded or supplemented. There has been much consideration of a range of other issues involved in marketing pharmaceuticals to physicians in the last few years and it is time to insist that the industry develop a more adequate and complete understanding of its ethical responsibility.

An issue of such fundamental importance, for example, as the extent to which the industry has been establishing financial ties with so many of the leaders in medicine needs to be addressed. The Washington Legal Foundation, an organization that does work in support of pharmaceutical industry interests, put it this way: "most of the top medical authorities in this country, and virtually all of the top speakers on medical topics, are employed in some capacity by one or more of the country's pharmaceutical companies. That is how it should be."[4] Is this really how it should be? The "how it should be" statement is a position about good medicine and good ethics that many would challenge. How can there be any realistic expectation of objectivity in medical education if so many of the potential speakers are in the industry's employ? It is important to make the point, as the Code does, that consultants and speakers should not be paid for work that they do not do, but it is even more important to protect medicine from the serious conflicts of interest involved in the pervasive ties between industry and medical "opinion leaders."

It sometimes takes a concerted effort to keep a discussion of marketing ethics focused on specific methods used in marketing the industry's products. The discussion can easily be sidetracked into a discussion of the value of the product and of the benefits that result from the use of the product. The fact that the pharmaceutical industry has contributed significantly to an improvement in the quality of healthcare through many of the medications developed and marketed should not prevent the public from demanding that tough issues be addressed. Even the most beneficial product can be promoted in inappropriate ways. The fact that physicians need information about new drugs and the pharmaceutical companies are able to provide information does not mean that the ways in which they "educate" meet the best ethical standards. It is not clear that statements like "Informational presentations and discussions by industry representatives and others speaking on behalf of a company provide valuable scientific and educational benefits" (section 2) belong in a code of ethics. Even if it is sometimes true, such claims should never be allowed to stop the conversation about the need for and the best ways to provide objective and unbiased information to physicians about the benefits and risks and cost of drugs.

The next three chapters are designed to contribute to a more complete understanding of the industry's responsibility by considering three practices involved in or related to marketing prescription drugs to healthcare professionals that are recognized but not addressed fully or adequately in the PhRMA Code: company-provided sample prescription medications; company-provided "educational" programs; and company financial support for continuing medical education.

PhRMA Code on Interactions with Healthcare Professionals

PREAMBLE

The Pharmaceutical Research and Manufacturers of America (PhRMA) represents research-based pharmaceutical and biotechnology companies. Our members develop and market new medicines to enable patients to live longer and healthier lives.

Ethical relationships with healthcare professionals are critical to our mission of helping patients by developing and marketing new medicines. An important part of achieving this mission is ensuring that healthcare professionals have the latest, most accurate information available regarding prescription medicines, which play an ever-increasing role in patient healthcare. This document focuses on our interactions with healthcare professionals that relate to the marketing of our products.

Effective marketing of medicines ensures that patients have access to the products they need and that the products are used correctly for maximum patient benefit. Our relationships with healthcare professionals are critical to achieving these goals because they enable us to—

- inform healthcare professionals about the benefits and risks of our products,
- provide scientific and educational information,
- support medical research and education, and
- obtain feedback and advice about our products through consultation with medical experts.

In interacting with the medical community, we are committed to following the highest ethical standards as well as all legal requirements. We are also concerned that our interactions with healthcare professionals not be perceived as inappropriate by patients or the public at large. This Code is to reinforce our intention that our interactions with healthcare professionals are to benefit patients and to enhance the practice of medicine. The Code is based on the principle that a healthcare professional's care of patients should be based, and should be perceived as being based, solely on each patient's medical needs and the healthcare professional's medical knowledge and experience.

Therefore, PhRMA adopts, effective July 1, 2002, the following voluntary Code on relationships with healthcare professionals. This Code addresses interactions with respect to marketed products and related pre-launch activities. It does not address relationships with clinical investigators relating to pre-approval studies.

PHRMA CODE ON INTERACTIONS WITH HEALTHCARE PROFESSIONALS

1. BASIS OF INTERACTIONS

Our relationships with healthcare professionals are intended to benefit patients and to enhance the practice of medicine. Interactions should be focused on informing healthcare professionals about products, providing scientific and educational information, and supporting medical research and education.

2. INFORMATIONAL PRESENTATIONS BY OR ON BEHALF OF A PHARMACEUTICAL COMPANY

Informational presentations and discussions by industry representatives and others speaking on behalf of a company provide valuable scientific and educational benefits. In connection with such presentations or discussions, occasional meals (but no entertainment/recreational events) may be offered so long as they: (a) are modest as judged by local standards; and (b) occur in a venue and manner conducive to informational communication and provide scientific or educational value. Inclusion of a healthcare professional's spouse or other guests is not appropriate. Offering "take-out" meals or meals to be eaten without a company representative being present (such as "dine & dash" programs) is not appropriate.

3. THIRD-PARTY EDUCATIONAL OR PROFESSIONAL MEETINGS

a. Continuing medical education (CME) or other third-party scientific and educational conferences or professional meetings can contribute to the improvement of patient care and therefore, financial support from companies is permissible. Since the giving of any subsidy directly to a healthcare professional by a company may be viewed as an inappropriate cash gift, any financial support should be given to the conference's sponsor which, in turn, can use the money to reduce the overall conference registration fee for all attendees. In addition, when companies underwrite medical conferences or meetings other than their own, responsibility for and control over the selection of content, faculty, educational methods, materials, and venue belongs to the organizers of the conferences or meetings in accordance with their guidelines.

b. Financial support should not be offered for the costs of travel, lodging, or other personal expenses of non-faculty healthcare professionals attending CME or other third-party scientific or educational conferences or professional meetings, either directly to the individuals attending the conference or indirectly to the conference's sponsor (except as set out in section 6 below). Similarly, funding should not be offered to compensate for the time spent by healthcare professionals attending the conference or meeting.

c. Financial support for meals or receptions may be provided to the CME sponsors who in turn can provide meals or receptions for all attendees. A company also may provide meals or receptions directly at such events if it complies with the sponsoring organization's guidelines. In either of the above situations, the meals or receptions should be modest and be conducive to discussion among faculty and attendees, and the amount of time at the meals or receptions should be clearly subordinate to the amount of time spent at the educational activities of the meeting.

d. A conference or meeting shall mean any activity, held at an appropriate location, where (a) the gathering is primarily dedicated, in both time and effort, to promoting objective scientific and educational activities and discourse (one or more educational presentations(s) should be the highlight of the gathering), and (b) the main incentive for bringing attendees together is to further their knowledge on the topic(s) being presented.

4. CONSULTANTS

a. It is appropriate for consultants who provide services to be offered reasonable compensation for those services and to be offered reimbursement for reasonable travel, lodging, and meal expenses incurred as part of providing those services. Compensation and reimbursement that would be inappropriate in other contexts can be acceptable for bona fide consultants in connection with their consulting arrangements. Token consulting or advisory arrangements should not be used to justify compensating health-care professionals for their time or their travel, lodging, and other out-of-pocket expenses. The following factors support the existence of a bona fide consulting arrangement (not all factors may be relevant to any particular arrangement):

- a written contract specifies the nature of the services to be provided and the basis for payment of those services;
- a legitimate need for the services has been clearly identified in advance of requesting the services and entering into arrangements with the prospective consultants;
- the criteria for selecting consultants are directly related to the identified purpose and the persons responsible for selecting the consultants have the expertise necessary to evaluate whether the particular healthcare professionals meet those criteria;
- the number of healthcare professionals retained is not greater than the number reasonably necessary to achieve the identified purpose;
- the retaining company maintains records concerning and makes appropriate use of the services provided by consultants;
- the venue and circumstances of any meeting with consultants are conducive to the consulting services and activities related to the services are the primary focus of the meeting, and any social or entertainment events are clearly subordinate in terms of time and emphasis.

b. It is not appropriate to pay honoraria or travel or lodging expenses to non-faculty and non-consultant attendees at company-sponsored meetings including attendees who participate in interactive sessions.

5. SPEAKER TRAINING MEETINGS

It is appropriate for healthcare professionals who participate in programs intended to recruit and train speakers for company sponsored speaker bureaus to be offered reasonable compensation for their time, considering the value of the type of services provided, and to be offered reimbursement for reasonable travel, lodging, and meal expenses, when (1) the participants receive extensive training on the company's drug products and on compliance with FDA regulatory requirements for communications about such products, (2) this training will result in the participants providing a valuable service to the company, and (3) the participants meet the criteria for consultants (as discussed in part 4.a above).

6. SCHOLARSHIPS AND EDUCATIONAL FUNDS

Financial assistance for scholarships or other educational funds to permit medical students, residents, fellows, and other healthcare professionals in training to attend carefully selected educational conferences may be offered so long as the selection of individuals who will receive the funds is made by the academic or training institution. "Carefully selected educational conferences" are generally defined as the major educational, scientific, or policy-making meetings of national, regional, or specialty medical associations.

7. EDUCATIONAL AND PRACTICE-RELATED ITEMS

a. Items primarily for the benefit of patients may be offered to healthcare professionals if they are not of substantial value ($100 or less). For example, an anatomical model for use in an examination room primarily involves a patient benefit, whereas a VCR or CD player does not. Items should not be offered on more than an occasional basis, even if each individual item is appropriate. Providing product samples for patient use in accordance with the Prescription Drug Marketing Act is acceptable.

b. Items of minimal value may be offered if they are primarily associated with a healthcare professional's practice (such as pens, notepads, and similar "reminder" items with company or product logos).

c. Items intended for the personal benefit of healthcare professionals (such as floral arrangements, artwork, music CDs or tickets to a sporting event) should not be offered.

d. Payments in cash or cash equivalents (such as gift certificates) should not be offered to healthcare professionals either directly or indirectly, except as compensation for bona fide services (as described in parts 4 and 5). Cash or equivalent payments of any kind create a potential appearance of impropriety or conflict of interest.

8. INDEPENDENCE OF DECISION MAKING

No grants, scholarships, subsidies, support, consulting contracts, or educational or practice related items should be provided or offered to a healthcare professional in exchange for prescribing products or for a commitment to continue prescribing products.

Nothing should be offered or provided in a manner or on conditions that would interfere with the independence of a healthcare professional's prescribing practices.

9. ADHERENCE TO CODE

Each member company is strongly encouraged to adopt procedures to assure adherence to this Code.[5]

6

Drug Samples: The Most Important Gifts

Central to the techniques used in marketing pharmaceuticals to healthcare professionals is the practice of providing samples of prescription drugs. Thousands of company sales representatives make frequent visits to physician offices and routinely leave samples of medications. Having them available in their offices, physicians can and do distribute these medications to patients. The practice is extensive. The retail value of the sample drugs distributed is estimated to have been $11 billion in 2001 alone, more than the amount spent on direct-to-consumer advertising and a major portion of the industry's enormous marketing budget.[2] One study found that these samples were given to patients in 20 percent of doctor-patient encounters.[3] Drug samples have been accurately called "the most important gifts" that sales representatives bring to physicians.[4]

The practice of providing physicians with sample medications has recently begun to be subjected to critical ethical analysis and assessment, but it does not yet receive the same scrutiny as many other practices involved in marketing drugs to physicians. In a national survey of physicians published in 2002, significantly more physicians acknowledged having accepted free drug samples from a drug company representative (92%) than acknowledged having accepted meals, tickets to entertainment, or free travel (61%).[5] Physicians generally find taking drug samples acceptable. The AMA ethical guidelines on what kinds of gifts physicians can accept from industry do not even address samples except in regard to the question of whether physicians may use these samples for personal or family use.[6] The "PhRMA Code on Interactions with Healthcare Professionals" identifies no concerns about this practice beyond the need to comply with federal regulations (section 7.a).

The major reason that the use of drug samples as a marketing technique has not raised many of the same concerns as other gifts that are given by company representatives is that it has often been viewed as a win/win/win situation. Many physicians like the availability of samples; many patients like to be given something free; the companies like having their products in doctors' offices. "The drug company increases awareness of its new drug. The doctor endears himself to patients by offering something of real value . . . And the patient can test out a new drug—which, after all, may not work or work well—without incurring any expense or even going to the pharmacy."[7] Further, the rationale often used to distinguish between acceptable and unacceptable gifts (discussed in the previous chapter) has clearly put samples in the category of acceptable. Because the distinction between gifts for patient benefit and gifts for the personal use of the physician is accepted as having key ethical significance, samples are not getting the careful scrutiny they need; they clearly can have a patient benefit use.

Providing drug samples is not, however, such an unquestionably beneficial practice. Not all stakeholders benefit. There has been growing recognition that, while the industry "wins," the practice does not promote high quality and affordable healthcare. A key concern is that the samples provided, because they are typically new drugs, are often more expensive than older drugs and, though approved by the FDA, may not yet have an established safety record at the recommended dosage. Companies have a financial interest in marketing their newer and most profitable products, which are usually those with patent protection against generic equivalents. The quick and widespread use of a new medication may be applauded at times, but new medications often raise questions about both safety and cost.

In the 2002 position paper on "Physician-Industry Relations," the American College of Physicians and the American Society of Internal Medicine acknowledged some of the problems associated with the practice of accepting drug samples from company representatives:

> The practice does allow the patient to try out a new medication before being committed to an expense. However, the sample serves to encourage physicians to prescribe the new product. Research shows that once a patient exhausts the free supply of medication, the physician typically writes a prescription for the same brand. Because few samples are for older or less expensive products, higher patient costs generally result. Moreover, physicians and their families and staff use approximately one-third of the samples, which illustrates how the practice fosters access to physicians' offices and encourages a gift relationship.[8]

Providing healthcare professionals with samples of prescription drugs needs to be examined carefully in terms of the overall impact of the practice on the quality and cost of healthcare and on the professional integrity of providers. Despite the widespread acceptance of drug samples, this marketing strategy should be subjected to the same critical scrutiny as other marketing practices used by companies in their efforts to get physicians to prescribe their medications.

ETHICS AND SAMPLES OF MEDICATIONS

In the past, much of the discussion of ethical issues related to sample drugs provided by drug companies focused on the use of these samples by physicians and members of their staff. While this concern continues to need attention (and is discussed briefly below), it is more important and more central to consider the potential impact on healthcare quality and cost when these samples are given to patients.

The practice of providing drug samples may contribute to the use of more expensive medications than necessary.

It is true that the use of samples sometimes saves some patients some money. It is one way in which physicians can help their low-income patients.[9] The samples from the office cabinet save pharmacy costs, a fact especially welcome to those patients who are without insurance for prescription drugs or those whose insurance requires a high co-pay. When the sample medication given to patients is a complete course of treatment, the availability of these samples means a definite savings for those individual patients. However, when the sample medications are just the start of a longer course of drug treatment, the patients who receive these free drugs may not benefit financially at all. The sample is likely to be a newer, more expensive medication, and, because it is available and free, it may be used where a less expensive drug is equally likely to be effective. And once patients are started on a medication, they will probably stay on that medication if there are no serious problems associated with taking it. The follow-up costs can quickly wipe out any initial savings for the recipient of a free drug. The "free" samples can end up costing patients more than if they had not gotten them.

The most important question about the relationship between free drug samples and the cost of healthcare is not, however, about the cost of medications to the individual patients who receive and use the samples. It is about whether the availability of samples contributes to the use by physicians of more expensive medications than necessary. Providing samples is marketing, pure and simple. It is not primarily assistance to patients with limited ability to pay for medications. Pharmaceutical companies do offer patient assistance programs, but it is important to recognize that the provision of samples needs to be reviewed as a marketing practice, nothing else. "Free" medications are offered to physicians to promote more widespread prescription of these medications. The true cost issue is the cost of healthcare across the board if and when the availability of samples leads to more widespread prescribing of more expensive medications when less costly ones are as safe and effective. The existence of samples in the doctor's office clearly makes it easier for physicians to prescribe them. "At the critical moment—the 'point-of-decision,' to quote the marketers' jargon—the drug is there, and it's free."[10] Once doctors have begun to use a medication, they are more likely to prescribe it in other cases.

Healthcare costs have been going up rapidly and, within these costs, spending on drugs has been one of the most rapidly rising components in recent years.[11] The cost of medications is an important ethical consideration primarily because there are limited financial resources available for healthcare. As employers, state governments, and individuals all try to keep healthcare costs under control, higher than necessary costs used in one area of healthcare mean there is less available to cover other needs. Higher than necessary cost thus becomes a threat to overall healthcare quality and accessibility.

Pharmaceutical companies claim that the use of newer medications improves health and saves healthcare money compared to the use of older drugs. Though more expensive, newer medications' greater effectiveness decreases the number and length of hospital stays.[12] This may well be true in the case of some breakthrough medications or drugs that are truly more effective than what was previously available. However, only a minority of newly approved drugs are significantly different from what is already on the market and the free drugs that are given to physicians are not just samples of truly innovative products. It is hard to dispute the claim made by Relman and Angell—that a genuinely important new drug does not need vigorous promotion by the company because physicians will get to know about such a drug very quickly.[13]

A variety of efforts are being made to limit increases in pharmaceutical costs. Managed care organizations have developed formularies of recommended drugs for physicians, based on both effectiveness and cost. They have introduced tiered co-pay systems for members to discourage use of more expensive drugs for which there is a comparable lower cost medication. More recently, a number of states have initiated vigorous efforts to control the costs of drugs in their Medicaid programs. "[I]n one of the more innovative programs, Oregon and 11 other states have joined in an ambitious effort to compare the safety and effectiveness of hundreds of drugs. Medicaid officials steer doctors and patients away from costly drugs found to have no proven clinical advantage over cheaper products."[14] These practices send the very important message that the cost of a medication, in addition to its medical appropriateness, should be a consideration when physicians make treatment decisions. This message has implications for the practice of providing physicians with drug samples.

Since pharmaceutical companies are in the healthcare business, their practices need to be assessed primarily in terms of their impact on health and healthcare. If there is good reason to think that the distribution of drug samples contributes to higher healthcare costs in the long run, the burden of proof is on those who would argue that these increased costs are essential to the improved quality of healthcare. (More discussion of the ethical significance of considering the costs of medications is found in chapter 10.)

The practice of providing samples may contribute to increased risks to patients.

The withdrawal of Vioxx from the market in 2004 has alerted a wider public to something known by the industry and by many physicians for a long time: there is still much that will be learned about the side effects of drugs and their interactions after they are marketed. While FDA approval means that a drug was judged sufficiently safe to be used and marketed, much more becomes known about the effects of the drug after it is used by many patients outside of the context of the clinical trial.

> When a new drug is first marketed, little is known about its safety and effectiveness compared to existing alternatives, and the situation is often no clearer years or decades later. We have a limited capacity to identify side effects early and reliably, and when a potentially fatal adverse event is detected it may take so long to enforce a recall that thousands of additional patients are put at risk.[15]

It is common that new dangers are discovered after drugs are already on the market. "According to a 1990 study by the U.S. General Accounting Office, 51% of approved drugs have serious adverse effects undetected before approval."[16] For many drugs, it is necessary to change the directions for use after the product has been on the market—usually to adjust the recommended dosage downward or to add warnings about risks to certain patients. Especially since the FDA approval time decreased following the 1992 Prescription Drug User Fee Act, the number of drugs recalled and the number that had a label change after approval has increased significantly. In drugs released from 1995–99, the corrections in the directions for use were, on an average, made three years after the drug came on the market.[17] Because of the unknowns, some doctors are wary of using medications on their patients until they have been available for several years.

Modern medicines tend to be very powerful interventions in biological processes. It should not be surprising that they often have other health consequences in addition to the intended ones. And some of these consequences will not be identified for some time after the medicine has been on the market. While this does not mean that powerful medicines should never be used, it does mean that the risks need to be understood as well as possible and that a medication should ordinarily not be used if there is something else less risky that addresses the health problem. The risks need to be managed. In Jerry Avorn's words, "Managing those dangers is becoming a central agenda for practitioners, manufacturers, and regulators."[18] Sometimes the drug's risks or dangers are proportionate to its benefits and sometimes they are not. Drug companies seek to provide physicians samples of the medications that they hope the physicians will prescribe more than they have been doing. Especially when the samples are of medications that do not yet have a long history on the market, the question of patient safety is particularly relevant.

It should also be noted that, even in cases where the physician gives a patient a sample medication that has a long history of use, there may be more risks with samples than with prescriptions that need to be filled at the pharmacy. When pharmacies are bypassed, there can be no safety check for drug interactions done by the pharmacist. It is possible, even likely, that, at times, providing sample medications contributes to unnecessary risks to patient safety.

Aggressive marketing may well increase the number of times that the benefits of the medication prescribed are not proportionate to the risks. The need to manage the dangers associated with the use of powerful medications has implications for all marketing practices, including the practice of providing free samples to physicians.

When physicians use sample drugs for themselves, staff, or families, they are accepting gifts for personal benefit.

Samples of prescription drugs are provided primarily to affect the prescribing practices of physicians. While most of the samples are used for patients, it is not unusual for physicians and office staff to use sample medications for themselves and their families.[19] The Prescription Drug Marketing Act permits the use of samples by physicians for themselves and their families and recognizes this use as conferring a benefit on physicians. The regulations accept this as an acceptable component of marketing the drugs.[20] When the AMA Council on Ethical and Judicial Affairs addressed the question of whether physicians may accept drug samples or other free pharmaceuticals for personal or family use, they took the position that this is permissible in certain circumstances—in emergencies, on a trial basis to assess tolerance, for the treatment of acute conditions requiring short-term use of inexpensive medications—but it "would not be acceptable for physicians to accept free pharmaceuticals for the long-term treatment of chronic conditions."[21]

When physicians—or staff—use sample medications for themselves or their families, these samples are best understood as personal benefits that are received from the companies, even if they were described as intended for patient use. In such cases, all the same considerations apply that were discussed earlier in regard to other gifts for the personal benefit of the provider (or staff); they may mean a serious conflict of interest. Personally benefiting from sample medications, like personally benefiting from other gifts, can compromise the physician's independence and objectivity. Gifts of greater value (e.g., long-term use or use of medications that would cost more out-of-pocket if acquired from a pharmacy) often have a higher potential for giving rise to a sense of indebtedness to the giver and, consequently, influencing and/or compromising behavior. Regarding sample medications, the PhRMA Code simply requires adherence to regulations governing the Prescription Drug Marketing Act, regulations which permit distribution for use by physicians and their families. A more adequate code would recognize the conflicts of interest that can result from such personal use and provide guidance on how to avoid placing physicians in these situations.

AN INDEPENDENT PERSPECTIVE

In this discussion, I have referred to samples of medications as being "offered" rather than as being "requested." It is true that the Prescription Drug Marketing Act requires that samples be provided only in response to a written request signed by a licensed practitioner. The regulations, however, permit the use of preprinted request forms.[22] In practice, the initiative in providing sample medications is commonly taken by the company, not by the physician, even though a request needs to be signed. It seems appropriate, therefore, to describe the process as "offering" sample medications.

Drug samples are the most important gifts provided to physicians by pharmaceutical company sales reps not only because of their large dollar value, but also because the samples are likely to have a significant impact on the practice of medicine. The responsibility for maintaining high professionalism in regard to the use of drug samples rests primarily with physicians themselves. The decision to accept and to use samples is theirs, not that of the company or the representative. The fact that samples are offered does not determine that they will be used or how they will be used. Nevertheless, it is an overly narrow view of ethics to conclude that companies that offer such samples have no responsibility about the consequences of their use. Making them available does not determine that they will be used, but it does facilitate, promote, and encourage their use and may contribute to their being used when they are not as appropriate as other treatment options in terms of safety and/or cost. The limited value of the PhRMA Code in recognizing and addressing the ways in which marketing practices can have negative effects is clearly revealed by its assumption that providing sample medications needs no serious ethical attention.

Because medicines are different from most other kinds of products, companies that manufacture and market medicines are not permitted to decide entirely for themselves when to put a product on the market and how to promote it. The FDA has the responsibility to oversee the industry and protect public safety. There is a growing belief that the current system for ensuring drug safety is not working. Companies play too large a role in evaluating the safety of their own products: "the major problem with the current system for ensuring the safety of medications is that drug manufacturers are largely responsible for collecting, evaluating, and reporting data from postmarketing studies of their own products."[23] The FDA sometimes requires, as a condition of approval of a drug, that certain additional studies be done after approval, but many of these studies are never completed and some are never even begun.[24] Physicians who observe adverse reactions to medications in their practice sometimes report these events to the drug companies, but "because of conflicts of interest or perhaps other reasons, some companies may neglect to fully acknowledge reports that indicate harm and fail to initiate proper studies to determine risk."[25] When companies have control over much of the data about the safety of their products after they have been approved, it is questionable whether the public is being adequately protected.

There is a need to change the system currently in place for protecting the public once drugs have been given initial FDA approval. Someone other than the companies themselves needs to play the key role of monitoring adverse reactions. Unfortunately, the FDA, as it currently functions, may not be the organization to do this best. Close ties exist between the FDA and the pharmaceutical companies and it is questionable how committed the very agency that approved a drug is "to actively seek evidence to prove itself wrong."[26] To have effective and trustworthy surveillance of the safety of drugs on the market, those assigned the responsibility to protect the public must be truly independent, free from organizational affiliations that might bias their work.

Just as independence is required for adequate drug safety monitoring and evaluation, so also is independence required for determining best ethical practices in marketing prescription drugs to healthcare professionals. Companies seeking to engage only in the best ethical practices in marketing their products need to acknowledge that, because of their belief in the benefits of their products and because of their interest in selling more products, they are not the best judges of their own marketing practices. Drug companies are not unique here. All companies believe in their products and all companies have an interest in selling more products. All companies have a bias when they judge their own marketing practices; drug companies are not different in this regard. Because of the differences between medicines and optional consumer products, however, it is particularly important to recognize and protect against this bias in the marketing of prescription drugs.

An independent assessment of the industry's responsibilities may be especially helpful in regard to the practice of providing free drug samples to healthcare professionals. Assuming that simple compliance with the Prescription Drug Marketing Act is all that is necessary to meet high standards of ethics is totally unsatisfactory. The failure of the PhRMA Code to address the serious questions raised by the practice of providing drug samples to physicians points out the need to continue the work to improve the industry's voluntary standards. An independent viewpoint may help.

Clearly, the least problematic use of samples is when the sample given is exactly what the physicians would have prescribed anyway, even if the sample were not available. This is most likely to happen when physicians request samples that are judged medically most appropriate, in terms of safety and efficacy, and most suited to their patients. It is not too much to expect that the pharmaceutical industry, if it is truly committed to promoting good healthcare through its marketing practices, will implement a true request system, one in which physicians will be provided only those sample medications that they have, on their own initiative and in advance, identified and requested. The ethical standards for marketing medications need to be higher than the ethical standards for marketing consumer products.

No one should rely on a business for impartial evaluation of a product it sells. . . . [T]here is an inherent conflict of interest between selling products and assessing them.[1]

7

Marketing Is Not Objective Education

Every year, practicing physicians receive a free copy of the *Physicians Desk Reference* (PDR), the reference that most of them make use of as a source of drug information. "Overall, doctors refer to the PDR 265,000,000 times a year."[2] The information in the PDR is written by drug companies and the companies support financially the distribution of free copies to 500,000 physicians, hospitals, and libraries.[3] The PDR is another of the gifts that the drug industry provides physicians.

The PDR contains useful information, most of it being the information contained in the package inserts that are distributed with drugs. It is essential to note, however, that the information in the PDR does not come from independent sources and that the free distribution every year effectively prevents independent references from competing successfully for physician attention and use. An independent drug reference might be expected to make "recommendations for selecting the best drugs and dosages for each clinical problem."[4] Such a comparison of different medications is not the kind of information provided in the PDR. The pharmaceutical industry cannot be held responsible for the failure of medicine to develop and distribute a better source of information on drug use, though its financial power and its influence might contribute to medicine's failure to do its own education better. The key point here is that the industry is the most important source of physician information about drugs.

The PDR is just one way in which the pharmaceutical industry provides information that practicing physicians have about the drugs they can prescribe. The industry also makes extensive use of clearly recognized marketing techniques: visits by sales representatives, exhibits at professional meetings, advertisements in medical journals, company-sponsored presentations. The industry usually describes these interactions with healthcare professionals as "educational." According to the PhRMA Code, "Informational presentations and discussions by industry representatives and others speaking on behalf of a company provide valuable scientific and educational benefits" (section 2). Critics of the ways in which the pharmaceutical industry influences the practice of medicine see the relationship between marketing products and educating physicians in a quite different way: the nature and purpose of marketing and the nature and purpose of education are essentially different. "[I]t is not really possible for companies to promote their drugs, which means touting only their favorable effects, and to provide impartial information, some of which might be unfavorable."[5]

John Abramson contends that, among the factors in the storm threatening American medicine, the most important, "the eye of the storm," is this: "the transformation of medical knowledge from a public good, measured by its potential to improve our health, into a commodity, measured by its commercial value."[6] In marketing drugs, with the emphasis on sales, the temptation is always to present primarily the kind of information that presents the product in the best possible light. In more objective medical education on drugs, the commercial emphasis is radically limited, encouraging an emphasis on the health benefits and the risks of the medication, usually with reference to other drugs and other options. Even though companies have an interest in being honest about the risks of a drug so that they keep physicians' trust, this does not remove the conflict between marketing and education.

There are other sources of information about medications available to physicians that are not ordinarily understood as marketing —such as articles in peer-reviewed medical journals, professional medical education programs (including Continuing Medical Education [CME] programs), and published clinical guidelines. These informational sources are provided by professional organizations and are generally thought to be quite separate from marketing. Even in these professional situations, however, there is concern about the independence and objectivity of authors and speakers. Most of the studies of medications that are published in the journals are sponsored by drug companies; CMEs are often supported by these companies, at least in part; writers of clinical guidelines are often consultants to the drug companies whose products they are evaluating. These concerns are addressed in other chapters. In this chapter the focus is on the responsibilities of the industry when it provides information on drugs to physicians in a marketing context.

CAVEAT EMPTOR

The PhRMA Code includes a section on informational presentations made by company representatives or others who speak on behalf of the company. The issues addressed are those related to the personal benefits that can be provided to physicians and their guests in this context: occasional meals, modest by local standards, are acceptable as long as they take place in a venue that is conducive to the informational nature of the meeting; company provision of a meal for the physician's guest is inappropriate (section 2). Given the concerns that have been raised by the industry's "wining and dining" of physicians, it is understandable that the focus of the Code in this section is on meals. The Code states, in the "preamble," that the professional's care of patients should be based "solely on each patient's medical needs and the healthcare professional's medical knowledge and experience." It should not be based, in other words, on the personal benefits that physicians receive. This emphasis is understandable, but it is not sufficient.

Limiting the personal benefits provided to physicians when selling drugs is a necessary component of marketing ethics, but it is not the most important ethical consideration related to these presentations and their impact. The most important issue, one that remains even if there are no perks whatsoever for physicians, is whether these programs are more likely to contribute to or to undermine good medicine. The ethical responsibility, therefore, is for the company to provide accurate and necessary information about the medications they are promoting—about the benefits and the risks and the appropriate use and the cost of these medications—and not to misrepresent them in any way. All those who contribute to the medical knowledge of healthcare professionals have a responsibility to reduce the risk that biased information will be presented (or received).

One way of focusing on the ethics of marketing and selling is to consider the question of what is owed to the potential buyer or consumer, a primary stakeholder. The answer to this question depends, in large part, upon the nature of the product and the risks associated with its use. Here we are considering the marketing of medicines, not some other kind of product, not some consumer good. The ethical standards for marketing prescription drugs need to be considerably higher than the standards for marketing products that are less essential and have less impact on the quality of someone's life.

Most of us are acutely aware that someone trying to sell us something has an incentive to be less than totally truthful about his or her product. One of the Latin phrases in common use in the United States is "caveat emptor"—let the buyer beware. If potential buyers are not attentive, they can be taken advantage of through the seller's use of exaggerations or half-truths, if not outright lies. In discussions of marketing, reference is made to "caveat emptor" for two different purposes. One use of the phrase is simply to acknowledge that consumers do need to be aware, to recognize the powerful incentive sellers have to complete the sale even if it means misrepresenting some aspect of the product. In this sense, "caveat emptor" reminds buyers that sellers may try to take unfair advantage of them. The other use of the phrase is to suggest that, when buyers are taken advantage of, it is their own fault; they should have known better. In this sense, "caveat emptor" puts most of the responsibility on the potential buyer.

In this second use, "caveat emptor" is sometimes understood

as a statement of the seller's lack of ethical responsibility: since buyers are responsible for protecting themselves, it is acceptable for sellers to use whatever techniques work to sell the product. Potential buyers should expect these efforts; they should protect themselves. Sellers do not need to be totally honest about what they are selling because buyers should not expect that of them. If this is ever a good standard of selling/marketing ethics (which is doubtful), it would seem to be so only in those situations: where the seller and the buyer both have similar access to full information about the product as well as similar ability to evaluate the information; and where there is no significant risk of harm to the buyer or anyone else if the buyer is taken advantage of. That is not the case in the marketing of prescription drugs.

In *Powerful Medicines,* Jerry Avorn writes of the benefits, risks, and costs of prescription drugs: "every drug is a triangle with three faces, representing the healing it can bring, the hazards it can inflict, and the economic impact of each."[7] As has long been recognized (consider the role and responsibility of the FDA), medications are not without the potential to do harm and their marketing requires careful oversight. Obviously, a whole different approach with regard to "caveat emptor" needs to be recognized as the ethical principle to be applied in marketing prescription drugs. A more appropriate principle is the recognition that pharmaceutical companies need to exercise "due care" to avoid harm.

The due care principle has been used most commonly to describe what the manufacturer owes to consumers who might be vulnerable to harm: "the manufacturer not only has a duty to deliver a product that lives up to the express and implied claims about it, but also has a duty to exercise due care to prevent others from being injured by the product."[8] It is useful to explore some of the implications, the ethical guidelines, that might result if a primary focus of the industry's code on marketing pharmaceuticals to physicians was on the responsibility to prevent users of these drugs from being harmed.

DUE CARE IN MARKETING

The standard for exercising due care in marketing prescription drugs to healthcare professionals requires a much higher commitment to truth than the mere avoidance of explicit deception. It means making available the information necessary for these professionals to acquire an accurate understanding of the safety, effectiveness, and appropriate use of the medications discussed. It means, furthermore, acknowledging that marketing and unbiased education are always in potential conflict and, therefore, that the company is probably not the best judge of how well it meets its responsibility to provide accurate and unbiased information.

This is a very high standard for marketing, needed because of the nature of the prescription medicines. The following are several possible implications of adhering to such a high standard.

Make the marketing nature of a company-sponsored program undeniably clear.

It is estimated that the pharmaceutical industry hosts hundreds of thousands of marketing meetings a year in the United States, meetings that they usually refer to as "educational."[9] When participating individuals are fully aware that the ultimate purpose of a particular "educational" program is to sell a product, they have a greater ability to keep themselves from accepting unquestionably the claims that are made. They can caution themselves to be more skeptical of what they hear in a marketing context than they would be if they were participating in a presentation made in, for example, a scientific context. They can remind themselves that the program sponsors and speakers have a clear incentive to present their product in the best possible light, an incentive that is in potential conflict with a commitment to complete accuracy.

Physicians need to be aware that company-sponsored programs are marketing occasions. Any and all speakers should be identified as representing the company. A featured speaker may be someone not immediately identified with the company, someone well known for research or clinical expertise. On this occasion, however, he or she is working for the company and should be presented as such. The reason for this emphasis is that there should be no misunderstanding. Good, scientifically sound information can and does sometimes get presented at company-sponsored programs for physicians. The context, however, is marketing, not education, not science. Education and science are being used, at least in part, to serve marketing goals. The commitment to educational objectivity can easily be subordinated to the goal of marketing the product. The appropriate response is skepticism: whatever information is presented will need to be verified elsewhere. (Given the tendency of researchers and medical journals to publish positive findings rather than negative ones, such verification is often not easy.)

One of the major reasons why it is important to remove or dramatically limit the personal inducements offered to physicians to take part in these meetings is that such inducements may incline physicians to be favorably disposed to company perspectives. A favorable disposition is inconsistent with the appropriate skepticism. Physicians prescribe drugs for use by patients and they are often paid for by a third party. Purchasers who are buying a product for themselves normally want to be sure that the product they are considering is right for the intended use and not excessively costly. Given the nature of drug prescribing and methods of paying for healthcare, this tendency is not fully at work here. The context is one of professionals listening to a presentation about a medical condition and how to treat it. To ensure the appropriate skepticism, attendees need to be very clear that those they are hearing, even if they are listening to physicians or researchers, are agents of the sellers.

It may seem strange to say that companies, in marketing their products, should be careful to remind physicians that the context is marketing. Doesn't this interfere with good marketing strategy? It might. Given the nature of the products that are being marketed, however, the public can legitimately demand that the marketing interests be subordinated to the standards of good medical science and good medical practice. To repeat a key point made in chapter 2, "prescription drugs are not like ordinary goods, and the market for drugs is not like other markets."[10] The ethical standards need to be higher.

Consider limiting radically the number of healthcare professionals who are part of the company's speaker bureau.

It is a common practice for pharmaceutical companies to have speaker bureaus comprised physicians and other healthcare professionals selected and trained by the companies to serve as speakers in their "educational" programs. The companies seek to employ in this capacity those academic researchers and others who have a good reputation among their colleagues and who are considered opinion leaders (those who give talks at professional meetings, contribute to textbooks, etc.). The "PhRMA Code on Interactions with Healthcare Professionals" identifies one issue related to speaker bureaus—the kinds of compensation and incentives that can appropriately be used to attract these professionals to serve in this capacity. The specific concerns addressed are whether the hiring and training of speakers is truly related to the services provided (their designation as speakers is not just a ruse for giving monetary gifts), whether the compensation is reasonable, and whether other personal benefits to the professional are limited and appropriate (section 5; see also section 4). These are important considerations, recognizing that any individual given special treatment by a company can have his or her scientific objectivity compromised. As was noted in the earlier discussion of conflicts of interest, there is always a real possibility that, even without any conscious awareness that it is occurring and against their intent, someone's opinions may be influenced by compensation and personal perks.

It is important for the industry code to address the question of personal benefits to speakers, though this might be one area in which the Code is open to the charge of being quite "permissive." The Q/A appended to the Code makes it clear that it is acceptable by industry standards to bring physicians/speakers to a two-day speaker-training program at a golf resort, which includes compensation for their participation, all expenses paid, and "a few hours" of company-provided golf (Q.i). While this type of compensation and entertainment might be considered reasonable in terms of the company's plans and expectations for speakers, it has the potential to undermine objectivity. And the potential impact on professional objectivity and integrity, not on what is reasonable in the industry, should be the key consideration.

There are other issues at stake in the use of a speaker bureau than those mentioned in the Code. There is a question of whether the whole practice of engaging many leading physicians as paid speakers in company-sponsored programs, or hiring them as consultants, may be harmful to the quality of healthcare. In 2002, *The New England Journal of Medicine* announced a questionable change in its policy related to the financial associations of authors who write review articles and editorials. The authors of these articles summarize data and draw conclusions; they do not report on specific studies. Freedom from conflicts of interest is essential in order to protect against the possible influence of commercial association on viewpoints that should be driven by scientific objectivity. The previous policy had been: "Because the essence of reviews and editorials is selection and interpretation of the literature, the *Journal* expects that authors of such articles will not have any financial interest in a company (or its competitor) that makes a product discussed in the article." The new policy changes "have any financial interest" to "any significant financial interest." The editorial board decided on the change because of the difficulty of recruiting authors for these articles under the former policy.[11] Financial relationships between pharmaceutical companies and physician experts are so widespread that it is hardly possible to find a reviewer who does not have some financial ties with the industry.

The New England Journal of Medicine described the policy change as a recognition that not all financial associations are the same; furthermore, it claimed that the change would allow it to be more successful in publishing important articles. The policy change also simply reflects the fact that financial ties between commercial interests and scientific medicine are ubiquitous. It might be seen, therefore, as an acknowledgement of the failure to keep the distance necessary for scientific objectivity. Good science and good medical education require independence and objectivity. The greater the extent of financial ties, the greater the threat to independence and objectivity.

Almost every time a controversy has arisen in recent years about the safety and/or effectiveness of a medication on the market (for example, the use of Zoloft as an antidepressant for children and adolescents), information surfaces on the financial ties of academic researchers to the companies making and marketing the drug. The public is being informed through news articles that

"Academic researchers routinely receive speaking and consulting fees from drug companies whose products they test."[12] Financial ties of this sort can, obviously, undermine confidence in medical research, in medical practice, and in the pharmaceutical industry. The problem is not that newspapers are making such reports; the public needs to know. The problem is not that some among the public may lose trust in medicine; losing trust seems to be a completely reasonable response to the reality. The problem is that these close ties established between industry and medicine exist and are allowed to continue.

In offering opportunities to physicians to make presentations at the request of the company, for a fee, a drug company is employing a strategy designed to increase sales of its products. In the process, it may be contributing to the breakdown of the distinction between scientific education and commercial marketing. It may be contributing, as well, to the decreased likelihood that medications generally will be subjected to impartial evaluation. There would be less likelihood that marketing will be confused with scientific education if clearly identified full-time employees of the company, rather than physician opinion leaders, were making the company-sponsored presentations. Reducing the size of the speaker bureau significantly may be one part of the effort needed to help restore the independence of medical scientists.

Provide the opportunity for healthcare professionals to review the results of all clinical trials of the medications being promoted.

In the FDA review in 2004 of the safety/risks of suicide related to the use of antidepressants (such as Zoloft, Paxil, and Prozac) by teenagers and younger children, one of the most significant points that came to light was that companies had not made public the results of some clinical trials showing a link between the drugs and suicidal behavior. The results had not been published in medical journals or made available in other ways.[13] The question of what information companies should make available about the results of the studies that they sponsor, regardless of the nature of the findings, is relevant to all other medications as well.

The appropriate standard is becoming increasing clear: it is not enough to present only the reports of benefits that might be expected from the use of the drug; the risks associated with the use of the medication must be presented as well. It is not enough to publish only the positive results of studies. Marketing medications ethically is not just about avoiding explicit deception in presenting the best possible rationale for prescribing the company's products. Good ethics also requires an accurate presentation of the risks or lack of benefits that may result when the drug is used. Because not all study results have always been made available to the FDA, it is not sufficient to simply repeat the warnings required by the FDA. For the sake of the patients, companies owe healthcare professionals easy access to the results of all clinical studies that have been done on the drugs that they are marketing, whether favorable or unfavorable to their product.

There has recently been increased demand for mandatory reporting of clinical trial results in a public database. This standard is supported by the AMA and the Association of American Medical Colleges. Congress may consider legislation requiring such reporting.[14] GlaxoSmithKline has agreed to post trial results as part of a settlement of a New York State suit charging fraud for failing to disclose the results of a clinical trial that showed no benefit in the use of Paxil.[15] Even if such disclosure is not legally mandated, the pharmaceutical industry owes the public, and those healthcare professionals who write prescriptions, accurate and timely reporting of the results of all the trials conducted to assess the safety and effectiveness of the medications they are marketing. All marketing directed at individual physicians should indicate exactly where and how to access this reported data. So should the PDR.

Make use of independent evaluations to prevent misrepresentation in the marketing use of published studies.

Perhaps because of the emphasis being placed on the practice of evidence-based medicine, pharmaceutical companies sometimes provide bibliographic references to published studies in their marketing to physicians (for example, in advertisements in medical journals).[16] Whenever they do this, they are making claims or suggesting a particular interpretation of study results. Given the incentive of the companies to sell their products, it is reasonable to wonder whether, in fact, the studies referred to really do support the claims made in marketing. One study of such marketing claims found that a most common misrepresentation is the (implied) claim that the drug is useful for patients different from those assessed in the study.

> Results from studies done in patients with specific characteristics (postinfarct, severe ventricular failure, etc.) had been automatically transferred to the population at large; alternatively, results were applied to specific categories of patients (diabetic patients, elderly people, women, patients with specific comorbidities) when these patients had in fact been excluded from the study (even when analysis of these subgroups had shown results that were not significantly different from the controls).[17]

Some misrepresentation may be knowing and deliberate distortion. Some misrepresentation may be less intentional. Regardless of whether the misrepresentation is deliberate or not, it is unethical advertising and has absolutely no place in the legitimate marketing of prescription drugs. Because all individuals and organizations are at risk of being biased with regard to their own practices, pharmaceutical companies that are committed to high ethical standards would do well to seek outside and independent assessment of the way they propose to refer to clinical studies in their marketing efforts. Before the use and effectiveness claims are made in marketing materials, outside and independent scientists—truly independent—should be asked to assess the legitimacy of these claims. It is not sufficient to wait for the FDA to intervene (the FDA does not review advertising claims in advance) and demand that misleading marketing be withdrawn. A responsible company will not simply rely upon its own self-interested review.

MARKETING IS NOT EDUCATION

Marketing prescription drugs is different from unbiased education about these drugs. By its very nature, marketing is much more an expression of the interest in selling the product than in providing an assessment of it. The fact that marketing is not education does not mean, however, that anything that meets marketing goals is ethically acceptable. The above four suggested ways of implementing a commitment to high ethical standards when marketing medications to healthcare professionals make it clear that the marketing of medications is not like the marketing of some other products. These recommendations are not the only important concerns that need attention, but they help make the point that marketing ethics is about much, much more than limiting the personal incentives to physicians. The ethics of marketing prescription drugs to healthcare professionals primarily has to do with the nature and the quality of the information presented.

"Medication decisions, while more reality-based than a century ago, are still heavily influenced by the triumph of hype and hope over data, of the politics of self-interest over coherent science-based policy."[18] It does not help that physicians get so much of their information about drugs from drug companies. Marketing, even when the types of suggestions made in this chapter are adopted, is not the framework for good scientific education.

Medical education, theoretically and presumably distinct from marketing, is itself at risk of being co-opted by commercial interests. This is the topic of the next chapter.

The drug companies pay the piper, and by one
means or another they call the tune; and the
tune is keyed to their sales pitch. The results
are clearly demonstrated by published studies
showing that industry sponsorship of CME is
usually followed by increased prescribing of
the sponsor's products.[1]

8

Medical Education: Industry at Arm's Length

It is a most interesting arrangement, one that many of the public
are unaware of and one that most physicians take for granted:
much of the CME that is required for physicians in order to
maintain their medical licenses is paid for by pharmaceutical
companies. CME is mandated for physicians in order to assure
that they remain up-to-date about developments in medicine. The
process for approving programs for CME credit is managed by
professional medical associations, and most of the CME presentations are made by medical experts, often from academic medical
centers. The role of industry in medical education is a troubling
one, given that commercial interests and educational interests do
not always coincide.

Commercial support for CME courses "has been increasing at
a rapid clip, doubling between 1996 and 2000. The medical industry (and in particular the drug companies) funded more than
three-fifths of doctors' continuing education in 2001."[2] The role
of industry in medical education is troubling because the interaction of pharmaceutical companies with physicians is primarily designed to get physicians to use particular prescription drugs more

extensively. Such marketing carries with it an enormous potential for incomplete or biased information. As noted in the last chapter, when people know they are the target of a sales pitch, they can remind themselves to remain skeptical about the information sent their way. Physicians who are seeking alternative non-commercial sources of information, ones that are more likely to be unbiased, may turn to articles in medical journals, CME programs, and clinical guidelines published by professional organizations for this information. Unless these professional sources of information are clearly separate from and independent of commercial interests, there is no assurance that they are unbiased. The professional and scientific integrity of the medical profession and its trustworthiness are directly related to this independence.

"As a learned profession, medicine has a fiduciary responsibility to patients in particular and to society in general to provide expert, unbiased advice on the use of drugs, based on the best available scientific information."[3] On-going education for physicians is the responsibility of the profession itself, through such organizations as medical schools, resident training programs, hospitals, and professional medical societies. Pharmaceutical companies are very different. Despite the fact that representatives of the pharmaceutical industry speak of both marketing programs and CMEs as "education," it is essential to insist upon the fundamental difference between product promotion and education. Medical education serves public health interests; marketing serves private commercial interests. Failure to keep the two separate and distinct risks the subordination of medicine to the interests of private companies. This acknowledgment of the important difference between medical education and the marketing of medicines is a necessary first step in identifying and understanding the ethical responsibilities of drug companies related to medical education.

One common method of protecting against the undue influence of commercial interests in medical education is to require that each speaker or author disclose any financial relationships that he or she has with the companies whose medications are being discussed. Disclosure does not, of course, eliminate bias or protect against conflicts of interest; it only alerts others that conflicts exist and that the potential for bias is present.

It is not at all clear how the non-expert, when alerted to the risk of bias, is going to be able to detect bias in a presentation by an expert. Another method of trying to protect the professional and scientific integrity of medical education is that providers of CMEs, not the corporate sponsors, select the faculty for CME presentations and insist that the sponsors have no control over the content of the program. This standard is important and valuable, but it is not always applied and, further, it does not address the more subtle influences that can result from the pervasive presence of industry money in medical education. The current protections are not adequate.

A key issue about professional sources of medical information is how to ensure that the content is not influenced by companies who have an interest in marketing their products. What kind of relationships between industry and researchers or educators are compatible with the need to have unbiased medical research and education? Maintaining the integrity of medical education is primarily the responsibility of the medical profession, but industry has important and essential responsibilities as well. Alan Holmer, of PhRMA, says that "the pharmaceutical industry is proud to play a leading role in sponsoring continuing medical education (CME) for physicians—an effort that serves the overriding mutual interest to ensure that patients receive the most up-to-date and appropriate care."[4] The pharmaceutical industry has, or should have, that overriding interest in appropriate patient care. This chapter explores the issues raised by industry involvement in medical education and suggests how that role needs to be changed if good patient care is to be put and kept first.

While industry also plays a role in the professional education of other healthcare professionals (such as pharmacists, nurses, physician assistants), the discussion here is focused on physician education. Many of the same considerations raised about industry and physician education are also relevant regarding education of other healthcare professionals.

CONTINUING MEDICAL EDUCATION

The Accreditation Council for Continuing Medical Education (ACCME) is the body responsible for setting the standards for

CMEs throughout the United States. In recent years, it has focused considerable attention on the question of how to maintain separation from the commercial interests that provide such a major portion of the financial support for CMEs. Providers of CMEs are often interested in accepting such financial support and usually accept it eagerly. There is presently limited money available from other sources and physicians have become used to the availability of free CME programs. The ACCME has been attempting to draw the lines that permit on-going support from industry while keeping financial support from leading to commercial bias or influence in the content of CME programs.

The 1992 "Standards for Commercial Support of Continuing Medical Education," still in effect in early 2005, do not address the issue successfully.[5] With the growing concern in more recent years about the influence of industry on medical education, it has become clear that the 1992 standards, in Arnold Relman's words, "leave much to be desired. They are permissive and ambiguous where they ought to be firm and clear."[6] The standards did not prevent ACCME from accrediting as CME providers many for-profit medical education companies that have pharmaceutical companies as clients,[7] and they did not prevent the council from accrediting some pharmaceutical companies as CME providers.[8] What some call collaboration between education and industry looks to others as the sell-out of education to commercial interests.

In 2004, the ACCME Board of Directors adopted the updated "Standards for Commercial Support," to go into effect in May 2005. As a sign of the times, these standards are subtitled "Standards to Ensure Independence in CME Activities," and the 1992 statement that commercial support from commercial organizations "can contribute significantly to the quality of CME activities" is not longer included.[9] The interest in collaboration (at least in terms of financial support) remains. The concern for protection against undue influence appears to have become a little more central.

The desire to ensure independence in CME activities may be more central, but the methods used to do this have changed only a little: commercial interests cannot "control" decisions about topics, content, persons involved; among those who are in a position to control the content, "all relevant financial relationships with any commercial interest" must be disclosed. The CME provider must have a mechanism in place to identify and resolve all conflicts of interest before the educational activity is delivered. In the process of revising the standards, a draft included the position that some conflicts of interest cannot be resolved by disclosure, that individuals with such conflicts should be excluded from participation as teacher or planner in CME activities. This tougher standard is not found in the final version. Unless the requirement for resolving conflicts of interest is implemented in a way that excludes those who have significant conflicts from participation in CMEs, these new standards also leave much to be desired.

As noted above, the position of PhRMA is that the pharmaceutical industry and medical educators have a mutual interest in CME.[10] There is some common interest, to be sure; pharmaceutical companies should be expected to have a major commitment to contribute to good patient care. But the fact that financial support for CMEs typically comes out a company's marketing budget does not suggest a clear recognition of the essential difference between marketing and educating. In subtitling its updated standards on industry financial support "Standards to Ensure Independence in CME Activities," the ACCME indicated its recognition that the drug industry's interests do pose a threat to the independence of medical education.

It is disappointing to many, however, that these updated standards still place a heavy emphasis on disclosure as a means of protecting independence. Disclosing a financial relationship with a pharmaceutical company does not prevent a CME planner or speaker from being biased. Instead, it is aimed at increasing awareness in the audience, most of whom are unable to detect bias even if they are more ready to look for it. Financial interests can influence people in ways that neither they nor others recognize. Studies indicate that a pharmaceutical company's support for a medical education program "was associated with an increased number of positive statements by CME speakers about the sponsoring company's drug and with an increased prescribing of the drug by attendees after the conference."[11] In view of the subtle ways in which conflicts of interest affect behavior, the insistence that commercial interests not be permitted to control explicit decisions about faculty and content, while a good point, may not be sufficient to protect against inappropriate influence. It remains to be seen whether the new standards will significantly change the extent to which CME is independent of commercial interests. Again, a key may be how the identified conflicts of interest are resolved. The continuing dependence of CME providers on industry money does not suggest a rigorous practice.

While the primary responsibility for maintaining the independence of medical education from commercial interests rests with professional medical educators, the industry has a clear role and an ethical responsibility in protecting this independence. If companies did not fund CME activities and if they did not employ academic physicians as speakers and consultants, the commercial threat to the independence of medical education would be significantly less and there would be fewer conflicts of interest. Being in the medicine business, drug companies have a clear responsibility to respect the integrity of medical science and of scientific education.

The "PhRMA Code on Interactions with Healthcare Professionals" does address the question of support for CME and other educational or professional meetings that are provided by third parties (section 3). As in other parts of the Code, the concerns addressed are relevant but too narrowly focused. The statements make clear, for example, that any financial support should be given to the conference sponsor, to reduce the cost to all attendees, not to individual healthcare professionals to cover their expenses or to compensate for time spent at the meeting. Industry provision of meals or receptions during a conference should be modest. These are important considerations. When healthcare professionals receive personal benefits from companies whose products they may use, these benefits can affect their objectivity when making decisions about the use of these products.

What is not addressed in the Code is the key question that the ACCME is wrestling with: how best to protect against industry support having an influence on the content of the educational program, how to protect the independence and objectivity of

CME activities. It is not enough to avoid putting individual professionals in the company's debt. As pharmaceutical companies and the public seek to understand the implications of the industry responsibility to respect and protect the quality and scientific integrity of medical education, the following standards should be given careful attention.

Pharmaceutical companies should avoid all direct and indirect provision of CME programs.

Holmer indicated that "A few pharmaceutical companies have been accredited by ACCME as CME providers."[12] It is difficult to understand how providing CMEs can be considered appropriate for companies that market their products so heavily to physicians. It is not reasonable to expect them to separate themselves from their commercial interests sufficiently to provide the kind of unbiased scientific education required, even if they make the effort to do so. An industry that considers the visits of sales representatives to physicians as "educational" even when they are paid to sell products is not in a position to provide unbiased scientific education. There is a clear and unacceptable conflict of interest when a drug company provides CME courses. The credibility of the ACCME is greatly diminished, if not completely destroyed, by the decision to accredit companies as CME providers. This is clearly at odds with any reasonable understanding of the ways to ensure independence in CME activities. Even if accredited by ACCME to present CMEs, though, responsible drug companies will avoid doing so. It is one thing for companies that make and market medical products to offer programs that are clearly recognized as part of the company's marketing efforts; it is something else entirely to attempt to present unbiased medical education.

Growing concern has been expressed in recent years about the role of Medical Education and Communication Companies (MECCs). These are for-profit companies, some accredited by ACCME, that prepare and present medical educational services, including in-hospital programs for staff ("grand rounds") and CME programs. The services are attractive to hospitals because they are organized by others and are made available at little or no cost. These services are paid for by the clients of MECCs, often pharmaceutical companies. Medical education is being offered to physicians, but it is being sold to drug companies. A report by Public Citizen, a non-profit, public interest organization, describes the role of these companies (called Medical Education Services Suppliers—MESSs—in that report) and some of the ways in which they promote their services to companies. It is clear that industry is being asked to pay for these services as a way of marketing their products. One MECC has marketed its services to industry this way: "Medical education is a powerful tool that can deliver your message to key audiences, and get those audiences to take action that benefits your product."[13] Jerome Kassirer reported a similar example of the way such companies try to sell medical education to pharmaceutical companies: "Very often doctors are more influenced by what other doctors say than what pharmaceutical companies have to say. So companies work through medical education companies to have doctors who support their products talk about their products in a favorable way. That's called medical education."[14]

Even if they are accredited to provide CMEs, MECCs that have drug companies as paying clients will inevitably be influenced by the desire to serve the interests of these clients. There is a fundamental conflict between having clients with commercial interests in the practice of medicine and providing unbiased medical education. Even if ACCME has accredited the MECC and even if the client company indicates that it wants nothing else than excellent professional education, the risk of bias is enormous. Accrediting MECCs is another example of the failure of ACCME to limit risks to the objectivity of medical education. But this failure does not excuse the pharmaceutical companies from recognizing their own responsibilities. The public should demand high standards of both.

Pharmaceutical companies should separate pharmaceutical marketing from CME.

Efforts are made in the PhRMA Code and in the ACCME "Standards for Commercial Support" to identify the appropriate use of the funds provided by companies to support medical education programs. This is necessary if and when industry financial support is accepted. The standards may, however, be more focused on the details of managing conflicts of interest rather than on the need to prevent them. For example, there is a stipulation about the kind of and location of commercial product advertising placement in the pages of CME content: "Advertisements and promotional materials may face the first and last pages of printed CME content as long as these materials are not related to the CME content they face *and* are not paid for by the commercial supporters of the CME activity."[15] This can easily strike one as missing the woods for the trees. Will conformity with this kind of standard really help protect the educational experience from undue commercial influence, especially while medical educators remain dependent upon industry money?

Much greater separation between industry and education is called for in order to protect the independence and integrity of medical education. Relman has said it well:

> If medicine wishes to continue as an autonomous profession, it should at least reclaim its full responsibility for CME. That means keeping the pharmaceutical industry at arm's length from professional education. Financial support from industry should be accepted by accredited educational providers only with the clear understanding that there will be suitable acknowledgement of support but no collaboration of any kind and no marketing links with the program.[16]

One suspects that the CME community is reluctant to keep industry at arm's length because it is fearful of losing industry financial support, on which it has come to rely. The pharmaceutical industry may indeed withdraw much of its support for medical education if the separation between education and marketing were insisted upon. It is not at all clear, however, that this result would be unfortunate. "Physicians may . . . have to pay more for CME but then may value it more, demand higher quality, and learn more from it."[17]

It is not part of the essential mission of the pharmaceutical industry that it provide financial support for medical education. There is no reason for the public to expect that. What the public can legitimately expect and demand of the industry is that it not use medical education as an opportunity for marketing. If the industry chooses to support medical education, it should be as an expression of its support for activities designed to promote the public good, not its marketing goals. To keep the industry's support at arm's length from medical education programs, no marketing links of any sort should be involved. This kind of support is more appropriately a part of a company's philanthropic efforts than of its marketing approach.

CLINICAL PRACTICE GUIDELINES, PROFESSIONAL ORGANIZATIONS, AND THE DRUG INDUSTRY

When the AMA launched a $645,000 campaign in 2001 to convince physicians not to take gifts from pharmaceutical companies, major funding for this effort came from a group of seven pharmaceutical companies.[18] How are we to understand this? Whatever else this joint venture meant, it seems clear that neither the AMA nor the drug industry recognized that conflict-of-interest concerns include much more than gifts; that all financial relationships between industry and medicine (including financial support for ethics education), should be scrutinized carefully. The industry may have become interested in recent years in breaking the pattern of gift-giving that many physicians had come to expect, but it clearly is not ceasing efforts to influence prescribing behavior. As Kassirer notes, there are other ways of influencing physicians:

> As the press has begun to write about financial conflicts in medicine and as the government has begun to promulgate rules about gifts, elegant dinners, and trips to fancy resorts, pharmaceutical companies have quietly switched their marketing strategies. They now try to influence the recommendations of practice guidelines developed by professional organizations with physicians financially connected to them who serve on clinical practice guideline committees and by supporting the organizations in other ways.[19]

Clinical practice guidelines can have a great influence on the practice of medicine. They are the statements, developed by expert clinicians, of the best current treatment recommendations regarding specific medical conditions. The writing of these guidelines is usually sponsored by a professional medical organization in that specialty area, such as the American Heart Association or the American Psychiatric Association. Practicing physicians, especially members of the sponsoring professional organization, are often familiar with and guided by these assessments and recommendations. Furthermore, these guidelines are sometimes used by managed care organizations when they identify benchmarks for the quality of care they expect of physicians affiliated with their plans.[20] These practice guidelines are a key component of physician education.

Given their significance, both practicing physicians and the public need to have confidence that the authors of these guidelines are indeed experts and that both they and the organizations that sponsor guideline writing are free from any financial and other interests that may reduce the authors' ability to be objective and independent. The present relationships between industry and medicine do not inspire this confidence; neither the writers nor the organizations appear to be free from serious conflicts of interest.

A major study of the relationship of the authors of clinical guidelines and the pharmaceutical industry published in 2002 found that 87 percent of the guideline authors who responded had some form of interaction with the drug industry, that 58 percent had received financial support for research, and that 38 percent had been employed as consultants or in some other way by a pharmaceutical company. Fifty-nine percent "had relationships with companies whose products were specifically considered or included in the guideline they authored."[21] Most of these authors stated that their financial relationships did not affect their own objectivity, though more believed it affected the objectivity of their coauthors. It is likely that they, like others, underestimate the extent to which these sorts of relationships affect their own judgments and actions.

Financial relationships between medical experts and the pharmaceutical industry are pervasive. As the chair of one guideline-writing panel said, "You can have the experts involved, or you could have people who are purists and impartial judges, but you don't have the expertise."[22] While this comment need not be taken literally (it is defensive and self-serving), there is little doubt that the industry has established financial relationships with many opinion leaders in medicine, a situation that leads to skepticism about the objectivity of clinical practice guidelines.

The conflicts go beyond those of individual authors. The professional organizations that initiate, sponsor, and publish the guidelines often receive major funding from industry, much of it actively solicited by the organizations. This funding, sometimes in the hundreds of thousands of dollars, can support meetings of the organization, publications, even operating funds, and, sometimes, logistical support for the writing of clinical practice guidelines.[23] When an organization becomes dependent upon industry money, there may be a sense of indebtedness to the donors. In addition, company representatives might well expect opportunity to be heard during the guideline-writing process. Similar to what happens with political campaign contributions, major financial supporters expect access in return.

In 2000, the American Heart Association's (AHA's) guidelines for the treatment of acute stroke upgraded the use of Activase, made by Genentech, from "optional" to "recommended" in treating ischemic strokes. A "subsequent independent investigation reported that six out of eight experts who supported the upgrade had financial ties to Genentech. In addition, contributions from Genentech to the AHA totaled $11 million between 1991 and 2001, including $2.5 million to help build the AHA's new headquarters in Dallas."[24] The financial ties may or may not have had an influence on the decision of the committee to recommend Activase. But they definitely raised the question of whether the recommendations were based on objective scientific assessment of the evidence or on other factors (whether conscious or not). As Kassirer noted, "We would not be asking these questions if the AHA had selected individuals with no financial arrangements with industry, or if they had not relied on huge donations from industry to support their programs."[25]

As the last quotation indicates, much of the responsibility for maintaining the integrity of the medical profession rests with the profession itself. Physicians have a responsibility to avoid conflicts of interest. The industry has responsibility, as well, to avoid the kinds of practices that place professional organizations and their members in these conflicts. The industry has a duty to avoid practices that have the potential to undermine the scientific and professional integrity of medicine. The translation of this general responsibility into practical standards and guidelines remains to be done, but a few initial suggestions can be made here.

Those who pay the piper call the tune. The only way to ensure that the tune, the clinical guidelines, is not called by the drug industry is to reduce the level and kind of their financial involvement. It would seem reasonable, as a starting point, for the industry to avoid altogether any financial support for the writing of clinical practice guidelines. That is a start in the effort to protect the integrity of that process, but it is not enough. Further, the level of financial support from pharmaceutical companies for professional medical organizations should be re-examined and guidelines that limit the size of grants need to be established. A grant or gift of any size has some potential to exert an influence, but larger amounts have a greater potential. The level should be low enough so that the organization's independence is not threatened, that the organization is not in any way dependent upon these grants. In addition, greatly restricting the number of medical experts who are employed as speakers and consultants is also important in assuring that experts who are not on the industry's payroll are available to author guidelines.

The public can legitimately expect the pharmaceutical industry to recognize the inadequacy of the PhRMA Code in relationship to medical education and develop much more adequate guidelines, making use of independent outside assistance in the process. Not everything that is legally acceptable is compatible with what pharmaceutical companies owe the public and healthcare professionals. The fact that medical educators and medical organizations seek their financial assistance does not mean that such support is appropriate. The consequences of permissive ethical standards that "allow an essential industry to put profits above the public interest are simply too grave."[26]

Physicians require on-going education about "the selection and discriminating use of the best and most cost-effective drugs—old and new, patented and generic."[27] The responsibility to provide this education rests with the profession itself. It is not the appropriate business of a marketing-driven industry.

> Medical research, even if it is conducted by the pharmaceutical industry, is not solely a commercial enterprise designed to maximize personal gain or company profits. The responsible conduct of medical research involves a social duty and a moral responsibility that transcends quarterly business plans or the changing of chief executive officers.[1]

9

Clinical Research and the Limits
of Commercial Interests

In an editorial in *JAMA*, Bruce Psaty and Drummond Rennie considered the ethical legitimacy of the decision on the part of a sponsor to stop a clinical trial before sufficient data were gathered to yield scientifically valid results. The early termination of a comparative investigation of different treatments for high blood pressure was the occasion for the editorial. No rationale except "business considerations" was given to the investigators by the sponsor for the decision to end the study early.

Psaty and Rennie recognize that, though drug companies are private businesses, "the recruitment and involvement of human research participants places clinical trials in a category decidedly distinct from the customary swapping and trading of ordinary goods and services."[2] Subjects volunteer to be involved in an undertaking which, though it may not provide benefit for themselves, is expected to benefit others through the contribution it makes to medical knowledge. An Institutional Review Board (IRB) that is doing its job well would not give approval for a research project involving human subjects to proceed without a reasonable expectation of scientifically valid results. Stopping the research prematurely prevents it from providing any useful medical information and thus breaks covenant with the volunteer participants; it exposes them to some risk without a justifying benefit of valid medical knowledge. The authors' argument is valid: "If the conduct of a seriously underpowered study is unethical, the willful creation of an underpowered study by the early stopping . . . seems unethical as well."[3] The legitimate reasons for stopping a clinical trial early include safety concerns and insufficient patient enrollment. These decisions should be made by an independent data and safety monitoring board (DSMB), not by the sponsors. In the case of the blood pressure trial, the DSMB recommended against stopping.

In undertaking clinical trials of medications, drug companies are engaged in a scientific undertaking, not just or primarily a commercial venture. Clinical drug trials, whether done by academic scientists or by private for-profit companies, are scientific studies and need to be conducted with a commitment to the ethical standards of research using human subjects and a commitment to scientific objectivity. In clinical research, both scientific integrity and protection of the rights of human subjects take priority over commercial interests.

In a 2004 study published in *JAMA* that received considerable news coverage, researchers reported that even "normal" blood pressure was risky in patients with coronary heart disease and that they can benefit from medication to lower their blood pressure further.[4] *The New York Times* article on the publication of this study is, perhaps, a signs of the times. The reporter not only described the study findings and the reactions of some medical experts but also pointed out that the study was sponsored by Pfizer, the company that makes a drug used in the study, and that the company saw the manuscript before it was submitted for publication. The story also included the statement that "Virtually all experts not employed by the government have been paid consultants for drug companies."[5] The objectivity of researchers, essential to good science, is not (or no longer) automatically assumed.

As more and more people become aware of the interactions between industry and researchers, these interactions are being subjected to critical analysis and review. An Associated Press story followed up the report of an expert panel on cholesterol guidelines with a story entitled "Doctors' Ties to Drug Firms Questioned."[6]

> Eight of the nine were making money from the companies whose cholesterol-lowering drugs they were urging upon million more Americans. Two own stock in them. Two others went to work for drug companies shortly after working on the guidelines. Another was a senior government scientist who moonlights for 10 companies and serves on one of their boards.[7]

The fundamental question is whose interests are being served by these financial and other ties. Practicing physicians and the public can have trust in scientific studies and literature reviews only if there are high standards to protect scientific objectivity and clear evidence that these standards are rigorously adhered to. This is not now the case.

Clinical research may not normally be included in the understanding of what constitutes "marketing" or of the ways in which the pharmaceutical companies seek to get healthcare professionals to prescribe their prescription drugs. It is included here, however, because company clinical research practices are closely related to their marketing interests. Publishing study results is one of the key ways in which industry seeks to influence physician perceptions and practices.

THREATS TO SCIENTIFIC INTEGRITY

Jerry Avorn has used the phrase "function follows funding" to describe the important influence of outside grants and contracts on the research agenda of academic medical centers.[8] This is just another expression of the perennial claim that those "who pay the piper call the tune" and the Watergate era advice to "follow the money." The source of funding is not the only factor to be considered in an analysis of the ethical issues related to clinical research, of course, but it is an important one. Even when a researcher would like to, it is very difficult to ignore or go against the interests of those whose funding provides the opportunity to do research, or the interests of those who are contributing to one's income, or the interests of those who may provide additional opportunities in the future. The sponsor's interests are powerful, even when not consciously embraced.

Some 70 percent of the money for clinical drug trials comes from the pharmaceutical industry.[9] It is reasonable, even necessary, to ask whether the fact that the sponsor is a private company that has a financial interest in the outcome harms the quality and integrity of the research. There are indications that this does sometimes occur. The two major threats to scientific integrity resulting from industrial support are bias and lack of openness.

Research support can lead "investigators, wittingly or unwittingly, to bias their findings in the companies' favor."[10] A systematic review of the impact of financial interests on medical research published in 2003 reached this conclusion: "Strong and consistent evidence shows that industry-sponsored research tends to draw pro-industry conclusions."[11] The examination of 1,140 studies found that industry-sponsored studies were "significantly more likely" to reach conclusions favorable to industry than those sponsored by others.[12] This is similar to the findings of other studies of the relationship of sponsors to the reported results.[13]

The reality of funding bias does not mean that all investigators are or will be biased by the funding source. Rather, it is an acknowledgment that, at times, "the financial association of authors with firms will skew the outcome of results in favor of the firm's interests."[14] Researchers may not identify explicitly with the sponsor's interests and may remain explicitly committed to objectivity. Nevertheless, the sponsor's interests can be favored, consciously or not, in the interpretation of the study results.[15]

The impact of sponsorship on scientific openness is both subtle and explicit. Contracts have sometimes required sponsor consent, or at least review, before publication of any study findings. Even without this contract language, there have been instances in which sponsoring companies suppressed or delayed publication of research results unfavorable to the sponsor's interests.[16] The explicit practice of requiring consent from the company is now recognized as so contrary to scientific ethics that it has few vocal supporters even among industry representatives. The appropriate nature of the sponsoring company's role regarding publication, however, has not yet been clearly determined.

In recent years pharmaceutical companies have sometimes farmed out the management of clinical trials to contract research organizations (CROs). These for-profit businesses provide a range of possible services including study design, site selection, statistical analysis, report writing, and preparation of the FDA application. CROs or the sponsoring companies may contract with site management organizations (SMOs) to manage the investigative site. These businesses may take responsibility for such tasks as negotiating contracts with investigators, acquiring IRB approval, and recruiting and enrolling patients.[17] At the same time, much of clinical research has been moving out of medical centers to other settings, with networks of community physicians being used to enroll patients.[18] CROs and SMOs have intensified the commercial pressures on clinical research since they have a business interest in pleasing drug companies, their clients.

There are a number of behaviors or practices or relationships present in clinical studies that are a matter of serious concern because they threaten the scientific validity or the objectivity of the study or because they put subject rights at risk. The following, while not a complete list, are examples of the concerns.

1. The sponsoring company designs the experiment in a way that favors positive results.

The triumph of commercial over scientific interests is reflected in studies designed to increase the likelihood that the results will be favorable to the company's product, even though the study results are misleading or have little scientific value or significance. There are different ways of doing this. (1) Studies sometimes test a drug against a placebo when the real question for good medicine is how the therapy compares with other available therapies. A study comparing a company's drug with a placebo allows the company, for example, to claim that a pain medication leads to "improved pain control" after surgery when the alternative in the study is no pain medication at all. The study reveals nothing at all about whether the drug studied leads to "improved pain control" compared with other pain medications already in use in post-surgery care. (2) Comparison studies can be rigged by comparing a higher dosage of the company's drug with a lower dosage of a competitor's product, or by comparing the company's product with a drug that is not a good fit for the symptoms. (3) Studies of side effects might test the product only on patients who are younger and fitter than the patients most likely to use it.[19]

2. The investigator doing the study has financial ties to the study's sponsor.

In addition to receiving project funding from a pharmaceutical company, an investigator sometimes has a personal financial relationship with the company as a paid consultant, as a paid speaker, or as a stockholder. Such financial interests are extensive. In academic medical centers, most of the experts who are qualified to direct a clinical study are on the payroll of one or more companies as speakers or consultants.[20] Despite the intent of the investigator to adhere to strict scientific standards, this conflict of interest carries with it a risk of compromise.

3. Subjects are paid or compensated for their participation in the research.

Sometimes patients are offered a fee for their participation in a research project or to compensate them for time and effort. Such payments raise questions about voluntary participation: Is a payment, especially a significant payment, an inappropriate inducement to participate? Does it make it too difficult for subjects to discontinue participation in the study once begun?

4. Physicians are paid to enroll patients in the study.

The incentives that companies provide to physicians to enroll patients in studies can be significant, up to several thousand dollars per patient enrolled. And sometimes bonuses are paid for reaching a quota of patients by a certain date.[21] The practice can provide an incentive for physicians to identify patients who are not fully appropriate candidates for the study and/or to misrepresent the nature of the study and its implications for the patient in order to secure consent to participate. It complicates a subject's decision to withdraw from a study once enrolled. If patients are aware of the payment to the physician, their relationship with that physician might change. If they are not made fully aware, their consent is not adequately informed. It is also doubtful that physicians who get paid large fees to enroll patients truly "earn" the money they are paid; a large fee for little work is the equivalent of a questionable personal gift.

5. Studies are stopped prematurely when there is no threat to the safety of subjects.

This practice was described at the beginning of the chapter. It needs to be addressed in comprehensive ethical standards for the conduct of clinical trials.

6. Researchers who write up the results of a study are not provided access to all the data.

The raw data from a study, often conducted simultaneously at a variety of sites, are collected and stored in a central location by the company or the CRO. Investigators may have access to only some of the data when they do their analysis.[22] Control over research data obviously has the potential to mean control of the analysis which, in turn, means control of the interpretation given in the published results. This threat to scientific independence and openness has been recognized as an important issue by editors of major medical journals, who issued a joint statement opposing research agreements that prevent investigators from examining the data independently. Lack of access to all the data of a study means that researchers and publishers may unknowingly be involved in misrepresenting study findings and thereby misleading practicing physicians and others about the effectiveness or safety of the medication studied.[23]

7. Experts not involved in the research are paid to be "authors" of the study results.
8. Ghostwriters are used to draft the original report of the clinical trial.

Thomas Bodenheimer refers to these two practices as the "non-writing author-nonauthor writer syndrome" or as the "guest-ghost syndrome."[24] The "ghostwriter" is usually an employee of the drug company or of a CRO or of a medical communications company who writes the article but is not listed as the author. The "guest author" is the expert who agrees to be listed as author of the study (and is paid for reviewing the manuscript). The expert guest author, selected to provide prestige, has not previously analyzed the data and did not write up the results, but reviews and has final control over the manuscript. This syndrome may be present in over 10 percent of published articles.[25] The risks here are obvious. Ghostwriters are not at all independent. Even if they are not told explicitly to report the study in a way favorable to the company's product, they know that the company will appreciate a favorable write-up of the study results. Guest authors maintain a theoretical independence. They have an option whether or not to play this role and they can approve of or revise the manuscript, but they have the incentive simply to edit the manuscript rather than to assure that the write-up is complete and objective.

9. Research results that do not support the use of the company's product are not made available.

As noted in chapter 7, the 2004 FDA review of the risks of suicide related to the use of antidepressants by teenagers and younger children revealed that companies had not made public the results of some clinical trials that showed a link between the drugs and suicidal behavior. The results had not been published in medical journals or made available in other ways.[26] This does not appear to be an isolated incident. A statement of the International Committee of Medical Journal Editors makes the point very clear: "Irrespective of their scientific interest, trial results that place financial interests at risk are particularly likely to remain unpublished and hidden from public view."[27] While there may be commercial reasons for withholding research information unfavorable to the sponsoring company's product, such a practice is clearly at odds with a commitment to good science and good medicine.

10. Contracts with investigators require review by the sponsor before any study results are published.

Companies that sponsor clinical studies often claim "ownership" of the entire database and seek to exercise some control over use of data. As noted above, contracts sometimes require sponsor consent and usually require sponsor review before publication of any study findings. The result is that some results do not get published at all and, in other cases, publication is long delayed. The question of data "ownership" and its implications requires much more attention. There is an inherent conflict between the ethical need for science to be open or transparent and the company's desire to protect proprietary interests.

11. Some "Phase IV research" is not done as a true scientific study but is conducted to get physicians and patients to use the drug.

Phases I, II, and III of clinical research include the various tests done to assess safety and effectiveness of drugs prior to approval by the FDA. Companies are sometimes interested in conducting additional studies after FDA approval, studies which are often called Phase IV clinical trials. Studies of drugs already on the market can be done to gather additional information about safety or to test for non-approved uses of the medication. Marcia Angell reports, however, that some Phase IV studies are surveillance studies of little scientific value: "sponsors pay doctors to put patients on drugs and answer a few questions about how they fared. There is no randomization and no comparison group, so it is impossible to draw any reliable conclusions."[28] Such studies appear to be nothing more than marketing under the pretext of science. The practice is an abuse of the scientific nature of clinical trials.

Given all of these threats to scientific integrity, it is understandable that John Abramson concluded: "In this commercial context, the age-old standards of good science are being quietly but radically weakened, and in some cases abandoned."[29]

STANDARDS TO PROTECT SCIENTIFIC INTEGRITY

Criticism of some of the interactions between industry and clinical researchers has led both the medical establishment and the pharmaceutical industry to clarify standards to be followed in order to protect scientific integrity. The industry response is best represented by the "PhRMA Principles on Conduct of Clinical Trials and Communication of Clinical Trial Results" approved in 2002.[30] Examples of the responses by leaders in the medical profession include the two-part statement of the Association of American Medical Colleges (AAMC) on "Protecting Subjects, Preserving Trust, Promoting Progress," published in 2001 and in 2002,[31] and the statement of the International Committee of Medical Journal Editors on clinical trial registration in 2004.[32]

The AAMC statement focuses on financial conflicts of interest in clinical research. The first part outlines policy and guidelines regarding the individual financial interests of clinical investigators; the second part focuses on principles and recommendations regarding the medical center's institutional financial interests. Two elements in the AAMC approach are particularly worthy of note. First, it clearly recognizes that institutional financial interests, not just those of individual investigators, can threaten the integrity of clinical research. This recognition, if taken seriously, should lead to a re-examination of the financial ties that presently exist between industry and the medical establishment. A second noteworthy component of the AAMC statement is the inclusion of the "rebuttable presumption" that individuals who hold a significant financial interest in a particular research project shall not conduct that research. Unless and until it is demonstrated that there are compelling reasons for doing so, these individuals will not be approved to conduct clinical research in which they have a significant financial interest. This principle challenges the belief that disclosure of conflicts is sufficient to protect against bias in clinical research. It will make a difference if widely accepted and if applied with rigor.

The policy adopted by the International Committee of Medical Journal Editors addresses a different issue in clinical research— the selective reporting of trials. The journal editors state that the ethical conduct of clinical research includes honest reporting. "Honest reporting begins with revealing the existence of all clinical trials, even those that reflect unfavorably on a research sponsor's product."[33] Selective reporting prevents patients, physicians, writers of clinical practice guidelines, and insurers from getting the full and true picture of a drug's effectiveness and safety. Beginning in 2005, therefore, these journals require, as a condition for consideration of a clinical study for publication, that the study was registered in a public trials registry before patients began to be enrolled. The intent is to provide incentive to register all trials. When all trials are registered publicly, "the many stakeholders in clinical research can explore the full range of clinical evidence."[34]

We can consider the PhRMA Principles within the context of these efforts by medical leaders to protect scientific integrity. The PhRMA Principles are divided into four sections: "Commitment to Protecting Research Participants," "Conduct of Clinical Trials," "Ensuring Objectivity in Research," and "Public Disclosure of Clinical Trial Results." While the whole statement merits careful review and is included at the end of this chapter, I will limit my comments here to parts of sections 3 and 4, the sections most directly relevant to the issues noted above.

Section 3, "Ensuring Objectivity in Research," begins with a strong statement of commitment to the independence of those involved in clinical research, in order to protect human subjects and "to ensure an objective and balanced interpretation of trial results." The corporate sponsors of the research "will not interfere with this independence." The specific principles that follow, however, do not always provide assurance that the industry recognizes the full implications of what is necessary to protect independence.

The PhRMA Principles acknowledge that clinical investigators or their immediate families should not have "a direct ownership interest in the specific pharmaceutical product being studied" (3.c), but they say nothing about an ownership interest in the company sponsoring the research. While the statement of principles is silent on this question, it is addressed in the Q/A appendix. In response to the question of whether a clinical investigator who owns stock in the company may be employed by that company to conduct the clinical trial, the response is: "Yes. Ownership of stock in the sponsoring company does not disqualify the investigator from participating in clinical research for the company" (appendix). Nothing is said about any limits to the amount of stock owned in order not to compromise objectivity and independence. Nothing is said about the need to report such ownership to the IRB or an institutional conflict-of-interest committee. Investigator ownership of stock in the company sponsoring the study that he or she is conducting appears, unfortunately, to be a non-issue for the industry. The industry needs to attend to this issue much more satisfactorily.

The issue of making additional payments for enrolling research participants is also addressed in section 3: "When enrollment is particularly challenging, reasonable additional payments may be made to compensate the clinical investigator or institution for time and effort spent on extra recruiting effort to enroll appropriate research participants" (3.c). It is understandable that, in a document like this, a general term like "reasonable" is used. But there is no recognition of the possible risks associated with such payments and no suggestion about who is to make the determination of "particularly challenging" and of "reasonable" or how these determinations are to be made. This statement permits fees for enrolling patients but gives no real ethical guidance. This opens the door to serious conflicts of interest.

Section 4, "Public Disclosure of Clinical Trial Results," appears to be almost as much an assertion of the prerogatives of the sponsoring company as it is a statement of its responsibilities. The subsection on "Sponsor Review" is an example:

> Sponsors have the right to review any manuscripts, presentations, or abstracts that originate from our studies or that utilize our data before they are submitted for publication or other means of communication. Sponsors commit to respond in a timely manner, and not suppress or veto publications or other appropriate means of communication (in rare cases it may be necessary to delay publication and/or communication for a short time to protect intellectual property). Where differences of opinion or interpretation of data exist, the parties should try to resolve them through appropriate scientific debate. (4.f)

The emphasis on "our" studies and data, together with other references in section 4 to the study database being "owned" by the sponsor, indicates a determination to assert control over the data. Those seeking reassurance that the drug industry respects the scientific values of openness and a commitment to the public interest are not likely to be satisfied. There is an acknowledgment of the very important principle that the sponsor will not suppress or veto any publication, but it is made in the context of asserting the right to review before publication. Taking a proprietary approach to scientific data in a document describing the industry's responsibilities in clinical research indicates that the industry is more committed to commercial interests than to scientific values.

Subsection 4.a, "Communication of Study Results," commits the sponsor to timely communication of "meaningful results of controlled clinical trials of marketed products or investigational products that are approved for marketing, regardless of outcome." This is a welcome commitment to providing the information necessary for doctors and others to make an informed evaluation of the risks and benefits of a medication. It is only a limited commitment, however. The same section states, "Sponsors do not commit . . . to make the designs of clinical trial protocols available at inception, as in a clinical trial registry." While the International Committee of Medical Journal Editors now considers such a registry necessary to have the full range of clinical evidence available, PhRMA companies did not commit to that in the Principles (published before the Editors took their stand). The industry's future responses to the new policy of these medical journal editors and to other demands for a public registry will reveal much about the nature and level of its commitment to open communication on clinical trials.

In the context of all of the serious ethical issues raised about clinical studies in the last decade, the PhRMA Principles are, at best, only a beginning. As in the PhRMA Code on marketing discussed in an earlier chapter, conflicts of interest are not adequately protected against. More important, there seems to be an incomplete acceptance of the fundamental principle that clinical drug trials, even when sponsored by for-profit companies, are scientific studies that need to be conducted with a full commitment to the ethical standards of scientific research. Much more attention needs to be given by the public as well as by industry to clarifying the sponsor's role and ethical responsibilities in conducting clinical trials.

PhRMA Principles on Conduct of Clinical Trials and Communication of Clinical Trial Results

PREAMBLE

The Pharmaceutical Research and Manufacturers of America (PhRMA) represents research-based pharmaceutical and biotechnology companies. Our members discover, develop, manufacture and market new medicines and vaccines to enable patients to live longer and healthier lives.

The development of new therapies to treat disease and improve quality of life is a long and complex process. A critical part of that process is clinical research, the study of a pharmaceutical product in humans (research participants). Clinical research involves both potential benefits and risks to the participants and to society at large. Investigational clinical research is conducted to answer specific questions, and some aspects of the therapeutic profile (benefits and risks) of the product(s) tested may not be fully known without study in humans. In sponsoring and conducting clinical research, PhRMA members place great importance on respecting and protecting the safety of research participants.

Principles for the conduct of clinical research are set forth in internationally recognized documents, such as the Declaration of Helsinki and the Guideline for Good Clinical Practice of the International Conference on Harmonization. The principles of these and similar reference standards are translated into legal requirements through laws and regulations enforced by national authorities such as the U.S. Food and Drug Administration. PhRMA members have always been committed, and remain committed, to sponsoring clinical research that fully complies with all legal and regulatory requirements.

Many different entities and individuals contribute to the safe and appropriate conduct of clinical research, including not only sponsoring companies but also regulatory agencies; investigative site staff and medical professionals who serve as clinical investigators; hospitals and other institutions where research is conducted; and institutional review boards and ethics committees (IRBs/ECs).

PhRMA adopts these voluntary principles to clarify our members' relationship with other individuals and entities involved in the clinical research process and to set forth the principles we follow.

The key issues addressed here are:

• Protecting Research Participants
• Conduct of Clinical Trials
• Ensuring Objectivity in Research
• Disclosure of Clinical Trial Results

These principles reinforce our commitment to the safety of research participants, and they provide guidance to address issues that bear on this commitment in the context of clinical trials that enroll research participants and are designed, conducted and sponsored by member companies.

1. COMMITMENT TO PROTECTING RESEARCH PARTICIPANTS

We conduct clinical research in a manner that recognizes the importance of protecting the safety of and respecting research participants. Our interactions with research participants, as well as with clinical investigators and the other persons and entities involved in clinical research, recognize this fundamental principle and reinforce the precautions established to protect research participants.

2. CONDUCT OF CLINICAL TRIALS

We conduct clinical trials in accordance with applicable laws and regulations, as well as locally recognized good clinical practice, wherever in the world clinical trials are undertaken. When conducting multi-national, multi-site trials, in both the industrialized and developing world, we follow standards based on the Guideline for Good Clinical Practice of the International Conference on Harmonization.

a. Clinical Trial Design.

Sponsors conduct clinical trials based on scientifically designed protocols, which balance potential risks to the research participant with the possible benefit to the participant and to society. Scientific, ethical, and clinical judgments must guide and support the design of the clinical trial, particularly those aspects directly affecting the research participants such as inclusion/exclusion criteria, endpoints, and choice of control, including active and/or placebo comparator.

b. Selection of Investigators.

Investigators are selected based on qualifications, training, research or clinical expertise in relevant fields, the potential to recruit research participants and ability to conduct trials in accordance with good clinical practices and applicable legal requirements.

c. Training of Investigators.

Investigators and their staff are trained on the clinical trial protocol, pharmaceutical product, and procedural issues associated with the conduct of the particular clinical trial.

d. IRB/EC Review.

Prior to commencement, each clinical trial is reviewed by an IRB/EC that has independent decision-making authority, and has the responsibility and authority to protect research participants.

- The IRB/EC has the right to disapprove, require changes, or approve the clinical trial before any participants are enrolled at the institution or investigative site for which it has responsibility.
- The IRB/EC is provided relevant information from prior studies, the clinical trial protocol, and any materials developed to inform potential participants about the proposed research.

e. Informed Consent.

We require that clinical investigators obtain and document informed consent, freely given without coercion, from all potential research participants.

- Potential research participants are to be adequately informed about potential benefits and risks, alternative procedures or treatments, nature and duration of the clinical trial, and provided the opportunity to ask questions about the study and receive answers from a qualified health care professional.
- Clinical investigators are encouraged to disclose to potential research participants during the informed consent process that the investigator and/or the institution is receiving payment for the conduct of the clinical trial.
- In those cases where research participants—for reasons such as age, illness, or injury—are incapable of giving their consent, the informed consent of a legally acceptable representative is required.
- Because participation in a clinical trial is voluntary, all research participants have the right to withdraw from continued participation in the clinical trial, at any time, without penalty or loss of benefits to which they are otherwise entitled.

f. Clinical Trial Monitoring.

Trials are monitored using appropriately trained and qualified individuals. The sponsor will have procedures for these individuals to report on the progress of the trial including possible scientific misconduct.

- •These individuals verify compliance with good clinical practices, including (but not limited to) adherence to the clinical trial protocol, enrollment of appropriate research participants, and the accuracy and complete reporting of clinical trial data.
- • If a sponsor learns that a clinical investigator is significantly deficient in any area, it will either work with the investigator to obtain compliance or discontinue the investigator's participation in the study, and notify the relevant authorities as required.

g. Ongoing Safety Monitoring.

All safety issues are tracked and monitored in order to understand the safety profile of the product under study. Significant new safety information will be shared promptly with the clinical investigators and any Data and Safety Monitoring Board or Committee (DSMB), and reported to regulatory authorities in accordance with applicable law.

h. Privacy and Confidentiality of Medical Information.

Sponsors respect the privacy rights of research participants and safeguard the confidentiality of their medical information in accordance with all applicable laws and regulations.

i. Quality Assurance.

Procedures are followed to ensure that trials are conducted in accordance with good clinical practices and that data are generated, documented and reported accurately and in compliance with all applicable requirements.

j. Clinical Trials Conducted in the Developing World.

When conducting clinical trials in the developing world, sponsors collaborate with investigators and seek to collaborate with other relevant parties such as local health authorities and host governments to address issues associated with the conduct of the proposed study and its follow-up.

3. ENSURING OBJECTIVITY IN RESEARCH

We respect the independence of the individuals and entities involved in the clinical research process, so that they can exercise their judgment for the purpose of protecting research participants and to ensure an objective and balanced interpretation of trial results. Our contracts and interactions with them will not interfere with this independence.

a. Independent Review and Safety Monitoring.

In certain studies, generally large, randomized, multi-site studies that evaluate interventions intended to prolong life or reduce risk of major adverse health outcome, the patients, investigators and the sponsor may each be blinded to the treatment each participant receives to avoid the introduction of bias into the study. In such cases, monitoring of interim study results and of new information from external sources by a DSMB may be appropriate to protect the welfare of the research participants. If a DSMB is established, its members should have varied expertise, including relevant fields of medicine, statistics, and bioethics. Sponsors help establish, and also respect, the independence of DSMBs.

- Clinical investigators participating in a clinical trial of a pharmaceutical product should not serve on a DSMB that is monitoring that trial. It is also not appropriate for such an investigator to serve on DSMBs monitoring other trials with the same product if knowledge accessed through the DSMB membership may influence his or her objectivity.
- A voting member of a DSMB should not have significant financial interests or other conflicts of interest that would preclude objective determinations. Employees of the sponsor may not serve as members of the DSMB, but may otherwise assist the DSMB in its evaluation of clinical trial data.

b. Payment to Research Participants.

Research participants provide a valuable service to society. They take time out of their daily lives and sometimes incur expenses associated with their participation in clinical trials. When payments are made to research participants:

- Any proposed payment should be reviewed and approved by an independent IRB/EC.
- Payment should be based on research participants' time and/or reimbursement for reasonable expenses incurred during their participation in a clinical trial, such as parking, travel, and lodging expenses.
- The nature and amount of compensation or any other benefit should be consistent with the principle of voluntary informed consent.

c. Payment to Clinical Investigators.

Payment to clinical investigators or their institutions should be reasonable and based on work performed by the investigator and the investigator's staff, not on any other consideration.

- A written contract or budgetary agreement should be in place, specifying the nature of the research services to be provided and the basis for payment for those services.
- Payment or compensation of any sort should not be tied to the outcome of clinical trials.
- Clinical investigators or their immediate family should not have a direct ownership interest in the specific pharmaceutical product being studied.
- Clinical investigators and institutions should not be compensated in company stock or stock options for work performed on individual clinical trials.
- When enrollment is particularly challenging, reasonable additional payments may be made to compensate the clinical investigator or institution for time and effort spent on extra recruiting effort to enroll appropriate research participants.
- When clinical investigators and their staff are required to travel to meetings in conjunction with a clinical trial, they may be compensated for their time and offered reimbursement for reasonable travel, lodging, and meal expenses. The venue and circumstances should be appropriate for the purpose of the meeting.

4. PUBLIC DISCLOSURE OF CLINICAL TRIAL RESULTS

Availability of clinical trial results in a timely manner is often critical to communicate important new information to the medical profession, patients and the public. We design and conduct clinical trials in an ethical and scientifically rigorous manner to determine the benefits, risks, and value of pharmaceutical products. As sponsors, we are responsible for receipt and verification of data from all research sites for the studies we conduct; we ensure the accuracy and integrity of the entire study database, which is owned by the sponsor.

a. Communication of Study Results.

Clinical trials may involve already marketed products and/or investigational products. We commit to timely communication of meaningful results of controlled clinical trials of marketed products or investigational products that are approved for marketing, regardless of outcome. Communication includes publication of a paper in a peer-reviewed medical journal, abstract submission with a poster or oral presentation at a scientific meeting, or making results public by other means.

- Some studies that sponsors conduct are of an exploratory nature (early-phase or post-marketing). These are often highly proprietary to the sponsoring company, and due to their limited statistical power, serve primarily to generate hypotheses for possible future trials. Sponsors do not commit to publish the results of every exploratory study performed, or to make the designs of clinical trial protocols available at inception, as in a clinical trial registry. If the information from an exploratory study is felt to be of significant medical importance, sponsors should work with the investigators to submit the data for publication.
- In all cases, the study results should be reported in an objective, accurate, balanced and complete manner, with a discussion of the strengths and limitations of the study.

b. Authorship.

Consistent with the International Committee of Medical Journal Editors and major journal guidelines for authorship, anyone who provides substantial contributions into the conception or design of a study, or data acquisition, or data analysis and interpretation: and writing or revising of the manuscript; and has final approval of the version to be published should receive appropriate recognition as an author or contributor when the manuscript is published. Conversely, individuals who do not contribute in the manner do not warrant authorship.

- Companies sometimes employ staff to help analyze and interpret data, and to produce manuscripts and presentations. Such personnel must act in conjunction with the investigator-author. Their contributions should be recognized appropriately in resulting publications—either as a named author, a contributor, or in acknowledgements depending on their level of contribution.
- All authors whether from within a sponsoring company or external, will be given the relevant statistical tables, figures, and reports needed to support the planned publication.

c. Related Publications.

For a multi-site clinical trial, analysis based on single-site data usually have significant statistical limitations, and frequently do not provide meaningful information for health care professionals or patients and therefore may not be supported by sponsors. Such reports should not precede and should always reference the primary presentation or paper of the entire study.

d. Investigator Access to Data and Review of Results.

As owners of the study database, sponsors have discretion to determine who will have access to the database. Generally, study databases are only made available to regulatory authorities. Individual investigators in multi-site clinical trials will have their own research participants' data, and will be provided the randomization code after the conclusion of the trial. Sponsors will make a summary of the study results available to investigators. In addition any investigator who participated in the conduct of a multi-site clinical trial will be able to review relevant statistical tables, figures, and reports for the entire study at the sponsor's facilities, or other mutually agreeable location.

e. Research Participant Communication.

Investigators are encouraged to communicate a summary of the trial results, as appropriate, to their research participants after conclusion of the trial.

f. Sponsor Review.

Sponsors have the right to review any manuscripts, presentations, or abstracts that originate from our studies or that utilize our data before they are submitted for publication or other means of communication. Sponsors commit to respond in a timely manner, and not suppress or veto publications or other appropriate means of communication (in rare cases it may be necessary to delay publication and/or communication for a short time to protect intellectual property). Where differences of opinion or interpretation of data exist, the parties should try to resolve them through appropriate scientific debate.

g. Provision of Clinical Trial Protocol for Journal Review.

If requested by a medical journal when reviewing a submitted manuscript for publication, the clinical trial sponsor will provide a synopsis of the clinical trial protocol and/or pre-specified plan for data analysis with the understanding that such documents are confidential and should be returned to the sponsor.[35]

PART THREE

MARKETING TO THE PUBLIC

10

Citizens and Consumers

Americans widely believe and are frequently told by political leaders that "we've got the best health care system in the world."[2] How good a country's healthcare system is can be determined, in part, by the health of the population. To measure a country's health, the World Health Organization (WHO) developed an indicator of "healthy life expectancy," which identifies the number of years that a child born now could expect to live in good health. The measure takes into account total life expectancy as well as expected years of illness. The healthy life expectancy of Americans ranks the United States 22nd out of 23 industrialized countries. Only the Czech Republic has a lower healthy life expectancy.[3] Other factors, such as the data accumulated in recent years on the large number of Americans who die each year because of medical mistakes[4] and the fact that well over 40 million U.S. citizens are without health insurance at any given time, also contribute to the doubts about how well the current healthcare system serves the American public.

The American healthcare system is by far the most expensive. The per capita healthcare expenditures in 2004 are estimated to be over $6,100, more than twice as much as other industrialized countries. "Even taking into account our higher per person gross domestic product, the United States spends 42 percent more on health care per person than would be expected, given spending on health care in other OECD nations."[5] It appears that many other countries are achieving better results and doing it at a lower price. In the words of Donald Barlett and James Steele, "Americans pay for a Hummer but get a Ford Escort."[6]

There are, of course, many areas of excellence in the U.S. healthcare system and many Americans receive excellent healthcare. But the system as a whole can definitely be improved. The presidential claim that we have the best healthcare system, quoted above, was followed by the statement that "we need to keep it that way."[7] Acknowledging that the system is not as good as it can be or should be is the starting point for seeking ways of improving present methods of providing that care, just as the claim that the system is the best can lead to protecting things the way they are.

Many factors affect the nature and quality of healthcare practices, including the methods of marketing healthcare products. In marketing prescription drugs, pharmaceutical companies have an obvious responsibility to the individual patients or consumers who use these drugs. The responsibility to the public, however, is not just to these individuals. Since marketing practices have the potential, even the likelihood, of having an impact on the nature, quality, and cost of healthcare generally, we also need to consider the implications of marketing practices for the system as a whole.

We, the public, are citizens as well as consumers. In Mark Sagoff's words, "We act as consumers to get what we want *for ourselves. We act as citizens to achieve what we think right or best for the community.*"[8] In acting as citizens, individuals work together with others for what they perceive to be the common good. This sometimes requires subordinating individual self-interests to the good of the community. Though a simplistic model of economic behavior suggests that individuals are only interested in their own personal and family financial self-interests, their participation in the community makes it clear that life is not so one-dimensional. Individuals often make decisions about their own consumer interests in a manner that reflects their concern for the well-being of the community as a whole, not just a concern for themselves. When individuals make decisions to buy higher-priced organically grown food, for example, they may do so because of a concern about the impact of "conventionally grown" food on their own health or they may be seeking to support a more environmentally sound model of agriculture. The growing interest in "socially responsible investment" indicates that many people want their money to support the kinds of businesses that they believe are socially beneficial at the same time that this money brings them a reasonable return. They are not simply seeking a maximized financial return. Even when acting as consumers, many are interested in more than their own self-interest narrowly understood.

A corporation that mass markets its products to the public is seeking to influence consumer behavior, but the advertising also affects others who are exposed to the marketing even if they are not interested in the products as possible consumer items for themselves. The public's knowledge and understanding can be affected, as well as their attitudes and beliefs. In mass advertising their medications, for example, drug companies can have an impact on the public's perception of what are normal imperfections or normal aging processes and what constitute problems needing medical interventions. Such advertising can affect general healthcare policy and practice in addition to the behavior of individuals. Marketing medical products to the public in an ethically responsible way requires, therefore, that explicit attention be paid to the potential impact on the public, not just on individual users of the products. The pharmaceutical industry owes the public the opportunity to exercise an informed citizenship role regarding healthcare as well as an informed patient role.

In this chapter, I introduce the topic of marketing prescription drugs to the public by reviewing some of the general ethical responsibilities that the pharmaceutical industry has to the public. In marketing to the public, drug companies owe patients/consumers and citizens (1) a recognition of and respect for the appropriate patient/consumer role in medication decisions; (2) clear, accurate, complete, and useful information on the benefits and risks of medications; and (3) clear, accurate, complete, and useful information on the cost of medications. These considerations will serve as a general background for discussing more specific issues and responsibilities involved in marketing to the public in the following chapters.

THE ROLE OF THE PATIENT/CONSUMER IN TREATMENT DECISIONS

Physicians and other direct care providers have traditionally referred to those receiving treatment, care, or consultation as "patients." Businesses who market their products for use by these individuals commonly refer to them as "consumers." The terms have different connotations and suggest a different understanding of the appropriate role of the patient/consumer in making medical treatment decisions. It is not necessary to argue for the exclusive use of either term. What is of fundamental ethical importance, however, is recognizing that "consumers" of medical products and services are not like consumers who buy clothes or a car or beer or even food. Industries that promote medications to the public need to do so in ways that recognize the specific nature of medications and the appropriate way that decisions about the use of medications should be made.

The current intense interest in medical ethics in the United States goes back to the 1960s. During the intervening decades, much of the ethics discussion and debate has been focused on patient rights. A brief review of the understanding of patient rights that has evolved can serve as a reminder of the appropriate role of the patient in medical decision-making and can help to clarify industry's responsibility to those who take prescription drugs.

The primary meaning of self-determination or autonomy in healthcare is that patients have the right to accept or decline proposed treatment and to choose from among proposed treatment options. The right of informed competent individuals to refuse unwanted treatment has rightfully become recognized as one of the most basic rights of patients in healthcare. Respect for human dignity and freedom means that patients will not be treated without their permission, that no medical intervention will be done without their consent. The whole "advance directive" movement, modifying state laws to allow individuals to make legally binding advance decisions about the medical treatment they will receive when no longer able to speak for themselves, is an outgrowth of the widespread importance attached to this consent requirement.

In order to exercise their informed consent role and responsibility, patients need to have good information. They need to be made aware, in an understandable and accurate presentation, of the benefits and risks associated with proposed treatment. Patients need to be provided the kind of information that reasonably conscientious persons require in order to make decisions that reflect their own beliefs and values. This includes information about medically acceptable treatment options. At least at times, patients require information about the cost of the treatment options as well.

At the same time that there has been this insistence upon the essential importance of respecting the patient's right to decide what treatment is acceptable, many ethicists have also been stressing the importance of recognizing the limits of patient rights. There is a difference between rights and wants; patients do not have a legitimate claim to whatever they want regarding medical treatment. Self-determination in healthcare does not mean that the patient is completely in charge of deciding what kind of healthcare is provided. There are different roles and functions for the treating clinician and for the patient. Physicians have a responsibility to use their professional training and experience to diagnose and make treatment recommendations. Physicians have a responsibility to proceed on the basis of the evidence available. It is the patient's role to accept or decline proposed treatment and to choose from among proposed treatment options. Self-determination does not mean that patients are permitted to prescribe for themselves.[9]

The discussion of "medical futility" has been helpful in highlighting the principle that the right to consent does not imply a right to demand. It is essential for good quality medical care to recognize that a patient should not get treatment that, on the basis of professional medical judgment, is recognized as having no reasonable likelihood of benefit. Treatment that is not medically appropriate should not be provided even if the patient requests or demands it.[10] In some businesses, it may be appropriate to see the customer as someone who is always right or to treat the consumer as sovereign. Healthcare is not that kind of business. Medical care is professional service. The responsibility of professionals is to provide recommendations and services based on professional standards and expertise. Medical professionals have a responsibility to practice good medicine. To provide patients with the treatment that they want simply because they want it (and can pay for it) is to confuse medical care with other services. Patients do not have a right to whatever medical treatment they want, if such treatment is not indicated.

This is not to say, of course, that the patient should be passive. Good healthcare requires that patients inform their physicians of their own insights into their health and that they challenge what they consider to be questionable diagnoses and prescriptions. But patients are not qualified to act as their own physicians. It is a misunderstanding of the meaning of patient self-determination for physicians to permit patients to make the determination of what is medically indicated or medically safe. The issue is not, of course, one of simply keeping roles clear. It is a healthcare quality issue.[11]

An additional clarification is useful here. In understanding the role of patients, the traditional distinction between therapy and enhancement is relevant. Therapy refers to efforts to cure or ameliorate a disease or an injury. Enhancement refers to efforts to improve performance or appearance when the person is already well.[12] Cosmetic or performance enhancement fits more appropriately into the category of "want" than of "need." It can be understood more as a consumer service than a healthcare service as traditionally understood. As will be discussed in chapter 12, the difference between therapy and enhancement, just as the distinction between medicine and consumer items, has implications for direct-to-consumer (DTC) advertising.

Most of the reflections on patient rights over the last generation have focused on the interactions between individual patients and medical professionals. This is understandable: it is in these interactions that the actual decisions about medical treatment are made. But these interactions do not take place in a vacuum. People enter them with different understandings and expectations that are often shaped by other factors in society and in the culture.

Understanding the nature and limits of patient rights has implications for industries that provide products used in medical care. DTC advertising frequently carries with it a suggestion about how patients should act in their interactions with medical professionals. Consumers are often told to "ask your doctor" about a particular medication. In assessing the impact of corporate activities and in seeking to implement best ethical practices, it is important to assess the potential impact of this and of other more subtle messages on the understanding of the role of the patient and of the role of the medical professional. The proper understanding of the patient's role is necessary to ensure quality and protect rights.

INFORMATION ON DRUG SAFETY AND EFFECTIVENESS

In the afterword to her book on drug companies, Marcia Angell suggests some questions that individuals might ask their physicians who suggest or prescribe a new drug. These include "What is the evidence that this drug is better than an alternative drug or some other approach to treatment?" "Is this drug better only because it is given at a higher dose? Would a cheaper drug be as effective if it were given at an equivalent dose?" "Are the benefits worth the side effects, the expense, and the risk of interactions with other drugs I take?"[13] It would be most interesting to observe how physicians react to these and similar questions. Even though they may only be asked occasionally, the questions are most legitimate. They alert physicians to the kind of information they should have at hand so that they, in turn, can inform patients.

Though a new prescription medication does not come on the market until it is approved by the FDA, it is usually the case that "little is known about its safety and effectiveness compared to existing alternatives."[14] The FDA does not require that all new medications be compared with other medications, only that they be effective in treating a condition (compared with a placebo) and that they be safe. "Safe" does not, of course, mean totally safe; it means sufficiently safe to be allowed on the market and used under the supervision of a physician. Medications, being powerful drugs, can be expected to have risks associated with their use. Some of these risks are discovered before FDA approval, but it is common that new risks are discovered after a drug has been approved for marketing and is in use. The use of prescription drugs has been growing over the last decade, with 40 percent of Americans taking at least one prescription drug and 17 percent taking three or more.[15] Since prescription drugs are so widespread in our culture and getting a prescription such a common part of visits to doctors' offices, it is easy to forget that drug use can be dangerous. In fact, prescription drug use can be very dangerous. Thousands of people die every year from the use of prescription drugs, many more than die from the use of street drugs.[16]

Whether something is sufficiently safe to use depends largely upon the benefits; to make a good judgment about risks requires good information about effectiveness or benefits. "The real question is whether a drug's dangers are in some acceptable proportion to the good it does."[17] The greater the health benefits, when compared to alternative treatment or non-treatment options, the more acceptable the risks.

A pharmaceutical company has a commercial interest in denying or playing down a medication's risks and in being slow to investigate potential risks fully. FDA regulations require it to state the risks that were identified at the time of approval (and any other risks that were later formally recognized by the FDA). When disclosure is not mandated, however, companies may be reluctant to act quickly on safety concerns that are raised about a medication, especially where millions of dollars are at risk. A company may be dedicated to safety, but there is a conflicting interest. The interest in sales works against the responsibility to investigate potential risks in order to provide the most accurate and most useful information to physicians and to the public. The case of Merck and Vioxx[18] is only one of the cases in which people have died using drugs while the company was slow to act on the mounting evidence of unacceptable risks. When there is no assurance that concern for safety and the need to inform take priority over commercial interests, there can be little confidence—and should be little confidence—in the drug industry.

The FDA requirements covering advertising to the public, described in the next chapter, constitute only the legal minimum. Companies seeking best ethical practices in marketing to the public will go beyond compliance with government regulations and focus on the nature of the public's need for information.

Drug companies owe it to the public to have and make available evidence showing how new drugs compare against drugs already in use to treat the same conditions. As noted above, whether a risk is acceptable or not depends upon whether the dangers associated with the use of that medication are proportionate to the good it does, to the health benefit that might be achieved. "For a given condition, some drugs are much better than others in their effectiveness, safety, and/or value for money."[19] A proper assessment of both the good that is reasonably expected from the use of the medication and the dangers associated with its use requires information on comparisons with alternative approaches to treatment. Without accurate information on how one drug compares with another drug or another type of treatment, a sound judgment about safety and effectiveness cannot be made.

Though the FDA does not routinely require such comparisons as a condition of approval, drugs for more serious diseases (cancer, for example) are usually tested in studies in which the control group is undergoing another form of treatment, not receiving a placebo. In these cases, it is considered a violation of research ethics to use a placebo with research subjects who have serious diseases if a reasonably effective treatment is already available. But for conditions like pain or high blood pressure or high cholesterol levels, placebo control groups are often used. This means that there is little or no mandated information on how well new drugs for these conditions, which are among the most widely prescribed and heavily marketed, compare with what is already on the market.[20]

To ensure that each new drug is compared with ones already available for treating that condition and to protect those companies from a competitive disadvantage when they want to do such tests and other companies do not, it is important to change FDA regulations through congressional legislation. At present the FDA can approve drugs that "offer trivial or no advantage over drugs already available, and may even be worse."[21] If approval standards required that a new drug be compared with a common treatment for that condition, both the new drugs and the useful information about them would likely be improved. When the drug companies themselves support such a proposed change, they send the message that they do, indeed, put their responsibility to the public above their marketing interests. Drug companies owe it to the public to support a change in the FDA regulations to require trials that compare new drugs with common treatment used for the same conditions.

Without easy access to clear and accurate information about the safety and effectiveness of one medication compared to others, the public is not able to make informed judgments or decisions. The public should be able to expect informed answers to the question, What is the evidence that this drug is better than an alternative drug or some other approach to treatment?

INFORMATION ON THE COST OF MEDICATIONS

One of the reasons for the growing criticism of the pharmaceutical industry in recent years is the increased cost of medications. The prices of individual medications are rising and the overall amount spent on prescription drugs continues to grow. Much of the public interest in securing prescription drug coverage under Medicare is a result of the recognition of how costly drugs have become for many seniors. Some U.S. citizens are importing medications from Canada and some state governments are aggressively seeking to obtain lower prices from drug companies for their Medicaid programs. Many individuals with private healthcare insurance have seen their co-payments for some or all prescription drugs increased. Individuals and insurers, both private and public, are all conscious of the increased cost of prescription drugs.

The issue is not just the cost of prescription medications by itself. Since 1995, the cost of medications has been rising faster than other healthcare costs and has been accompanied by pharmaceutical industry profits that are consistently higher than those of almost all other industries.[22] DTC advertising, almost all of which is for newer higher-priced medications, has increased enormously in recent years. Furthermore, the public is becoming aware of the ways in which the industry has taken advantage of "loopholes" in patent laws to extend the period of time before lower-priced generics are marketed.[23] And the new drugs being marketed are frequently "me-too" drugs, similar to what is already on the market instead of innovative treatments. Prescription drugs "in the United States cost from 30 percent to 60 percent more than the exact same medications sold anywhere else in the industrialized world."[24] The industry, which has an extensive lobbying force in Washington and has contributed heavily to political campaigns, is expected to achieve further financial benefits from the recently enacted Medicare prescription drug benefit program which prohibits the federal government from negotiating discounts from the drug companies.[25] All of this has led many to ask whether the public is being exploited and whether medications are worth the cost.

Representatives from pharmaceutical companies often point out that the amount of money spent on prescription drugs is only a small part of the total healthcare bill in the United States— roughly 10 percent.[26] This point can serve as an important reminder that addressing the costs of drugs will clearly not resolve all the issues associated with healthcare costs. Nevertheless, there are good reasons for focusing on the cost of drugs. Many other expenditures have fixed costs associated with them (hospitals and laboratories need to be staffed, for example), while medications do not have similar fixed costs.[27] Furthermore, the increasing cost of prescription drugs has occurred at a time of aggressive advertising of these drugs to the public. Perhaps even more important, there is increasing evidence that refraining from the use of some costly drugs "can keep expenditures in check without any clinical downsides" because they are no better than less expensive treatments.[28]

The real issue, of course, is whether a particular drug is worth the cost—whether it is needed and whether it is better than less expensive alternatives. Do the drugs prescribed represent high-quality and cost-effective medical treatment? Not all prescriptions are equally good medical decisions and not all are equally good use of money: "some medications are great buys that produce substantial medical benefit for a modest cost; others are bad deals that consume many dollars while providing little or no health benefit in return."[29] A commitment to improved quality in healthcare is fully compatible with a commitment to cost sensitivity in the use of medications. Sometimes, the less expensive medication provides results that are just as good, with a lower risk of serious side effects.[30] The issue is not just the overall cost of medications but also the benefits, risks, and costs of specific medications.

It is important to continue to emphasize that medical drugs are not like consumer items. If, influenced by marketing techniques, I buy a computer that does not meet my needs, I am not putting my health at risk. If it is more expensive than I need, I am not likely to be depriving others of a chance to use a computer. If I take medications that do not fit my needs, I may be harmed unnecessarily (even if unintentionally) and/or I may be placing an unnecessary burden on finite shared healthcare resources, thus limiting the healthcare resources available to others to receive needed healthcare. And when companies market their products aggressively, the responsibility for this harm and this waste of limited resources rests with the companies that influence the prescription decision as well as with the prescribing physician. Marketing medications is different, ethically, from marketing optional consumer items.

The public needs easy access to clear, accurate, and useful information about the cost of specific medications. Patients have a right to know, and a need to know, the cost of medications prescribed. How else can they be assured that a particular medication is worth the cost? One of the questions that Angell suggests that patients ask their doctors is "Are the benefits worth the side effects, the expense, and the risk of interaction with other drugs I take?"[31] As discussed above, patients/consumers generally do not have the training and competence necessary to decide what kind of treatment is medically appropriate. But they do have responsibility to decide whether the treatment recommended is acceptable. And they can/should demand that physicians take cost into account, as well as possible benefits and risks. If different medications are available to treat a specific condition, many consumers will want to know, and citizens need to know, which "are better than others in their effectiveness, safety, and/or value for money."[32] The question about cost, it is important to emphasize, is not just what this is going to cost me, as an individual consumer, out of my own pocket. The cost, even when covered by insurance, remains a very important consideration for those who are interested in containing the cost of medicine and using resources wisely.

Patients depend upon their physicians to know about a medication's effectiveness and safety. Even though, as has been discussed in earlier chapters, the information provided to physicians through journal articles, continuing medical education, and marketing is sometimes incomplete or misleading, patients are not in a position to assess effectiveness and safety themselves. They do need to depend upon physicians, using pointed questions, perhaps, to push physicians to explain why they are choosing one medication rather than another. Many physicians are notoriously unaware of the cost of the treatment that they prescribe or recommend, however, so patients cannot presently depend upon them for accurate and comparative information on costs. If patients are insured, their healthcare plan may well have guidelines or formularies that seek to bring cost-effectiveness considerations into the process of writing prescriptions. That information, however, is not normally provided to patients themselves. It is not easy for a patient to have the information available to determine whether a particular medication is worth the cost.

In their role as citizens, perhaps even more than in their role as patients/consumers, the public needs to know the cost of different medications. The Medicare Act of 2003 prohibited the federal government from setting or negotiating the prices it pays for the drugs covered by Medicare. This is most unusual, indeed incomprehensible. The Medicare program does not permit hospitals or physicians to set their own prices for Medicare patients. Nor does the federal government permit an aircraft company "to put whatever price tag it wanted on the latest jet fighter it was selling to the Air Force."[33] Ordinarily, when a decision is made that something is so necessary for the public good that it must be provided by the federal government, the government requires bids or otherwise determines/negotiates what it will pay for different services. Part of the explanation for the decision not to do this in Medicare prescription drug coverage is the political clout of the pharmaceutical industry. Perhaps a part of the explanation as well is that the public is not yet adequately informed about the comparative costs and comparative risks and benefits of different medications for treating the same conditions. Without a greater recognition regarding which medications are "great buys that produce substantial medical benefit for a modest cost" and which are "bad deals that consume many dollars while providing little or no health benefit,"[34] it might be easy to accept the marketing claims about new medications and fail to demand that the real value (in terms of benefits and costs) needs to be proven.

The organizational self-interest of pharmaceutical companies in selling their most profitable medications may contribute unnecessary costs and may harm the healthcare system and those served by it. The industry does not contribute to an adequately informed public unless it provides accurate information on comparative cost as well as accurate information on comparative effectiveness and risks. In order to move the American system in the direction of "the best health care system in the world," the public needs to insist that this information be made available.

> On a scale no one could have foreseen, the drug companies have enlisted the expertise of Madison Avenue to sell . . . their wares. Using techniques advertising has perfected over decades to entice consumers to buy soap, cereal, beer, perfume, and dog food, the drug companies are transforming the way we look at medicines.[1]

11

Direct-to-Consumer Advertising:
Conflicting Interests

In December, 2004, Pfizer suspended its advertising of the pain reliever Celebrex on radio, on TV, in newspapers, and in magazines. This decision, made in conversations with the FDA, followed the release of study results which suggested an increased risk of heart attacks in patients who took high dosages of Celebrex. Pfizer's decision on DTC advertising did not include a decision to withdraw Celebrex from the market or to terminate marketing Celebrex to physicians.[2]

The decision struck some as strange. In the words of one letter-to-the-editor writer, the decision to refrain from using mass marketing advertising for a product that the company stills considers safe and effective when properly used is a decision that "strains logic." If it is truly safe and effective, the company has "little to fear from advertising it to the public." Stopping mass advertising while keeping the product on the market "will only foster the public's growing perception that the drug companies place profit ahead of public safety."[3] The public will read this decision, presumably, as a recognition that Celebrex is dangerous but Pfizer wants to continue to sell it anyway.

There is another and quite different way of viewing this decision. The decision can be seen as a recognition that there is a difference between (1) approving a medication as sufficiently safe and effective to be used for some patients and (2) advertising that medication to millions of people through the techniques of mass media product promotion. It is one thing to make a medication available for use if, in the judgment of an informed physician, it is the best treatment for the condition and the benefits outweigh the risks in a particular case. It is something very different to encourage everyone who watches TV to "ask your doctor" if this medication is "right for you" if you have any aches or pains. The decision not to continue DTC advertising of Celebrex while recent studies on the drug's side effects are being evaluated could be read as an implicit acknowledgment that DTC advertising has the potential to contribute to unnecessary and/or excessive use of medications that are fully appropriate in some cases.

The United States stands almost alone in permitting the DTC advertising of prescription drugs; New Zealand is the only other country that does.[4] Elsewhere, the prevailing belief is that the disadvantages or harm to the public health of such advertising outweigh the advantages or benefits—and there are many in the United States and in New Zealand who agree with that judgment. Such ads may seem to be a part of the American way of life, but they are a very recent development and the effects on public health are very much in dispute. It is only since the FDA policy change in 1997 that DTC advertising, especially on TV, has increased dramatically. In that year, the FDA introduced more permissive regulations for TV and radio advertising of prescription drugs, permitting such advertising without the kind of detailed medical information on risks and side effects still found in print advertising (in the small print). Only major side effects and major contraindications need to be mentioned in broadcast ads, along with a reference to a location where more detailed information can be found.

Spending on DTC advertising has been increasing rapidly, up to $3 billion already in 2001.[5] The most heavily advertised drugs are for treatment of such conditions as arthritis, ulcers, allergies, depression, high cholesterol, sexual dysfunction, and asthma. It is not surprising that most of the spending on DTC advertising is for drugs used to treat chronic illnesses or conditions/symptoms that afflict millions of Americans, because these are the drugs that have very large potential markets.[6] Sales of the most heavily advertised drugs rose faster than those not heavily advertised to consumers,[7] and DTC advertising increased sales within each drug's class. For example, advertising for one antihistamine meant increased sales for other antihistamines as well as the one advertised.[8] DTC advertising has a significant "payoff" for the industry: "every additional $1 the industry spent on DTC advertising in 2000 yielded an additional $4.20 in sales."[9] Whether DTC advertising "pays off" in terms of public health is strenuously debated.[10]

The FDA has responsibility to regulate advertising of prescription drugs, including the responsibility to assure that the content of ads is accurate and represents fairly both the benefits and the risks. Companies need to submit all drug ads to the FDA when they are first disseminated to the public, but they do not need specific FDA approval of an ad in advance (unless the drug was approved on an accelerated basis).[11] The FDA has authority to issue letters to companies demanding that misleading ads be withdrawn, but this is often done after the ads have been broadcast for months.[12] Sometimes the same companies need to be sent letters about misleading ads for the same drug: the "FDA has issued four regulatory letters to Pfizer regarding broadcast and print advertisements for its cholesterol-lowering drug, Lipitor. Among other infractions, FDA noted that the advertisements gave the false impression that Lipitor can reduce heart disease and falsely claimed that Lipitor is safer than competing products."[13] Letters bring compliance in specific cases but do not provide assurance that other misleading ads will not follow and be disseminated widely before being withdrawn.

The FDA recognizes three types of DTC ads: help-seeking or disease-oriented ads; reminder ads; and product-claim ads. (1) Help-seeking ads are those that "typically describe the symptoms of a disease or condition, and encourage consumers to consult their physicians to discuss treatment options."[14] A particular drug is not identified, but the company sponsoring the ad is identified. (2) Reminder ads use the name of the drug but do not include the disease or condition to be treated and do not provide information about the product. These are used to build brand-name recognition. They also encourage consumers to see their doctor. Reminder ads do not need to contain detailed information about the drug's effectiveness or potential side effects, though the FDA does not permit drugs that need to carry a "black box" warning (the method used to emphasize a warning of potential serious side effects) to be promoted through reminder ads. (3) Product-claim ads include both the drug's brand name and its intended use. Consumers who may have a specific condition are urged to ask their doctors about a specific drug. The FDA rules for product-claim ads require a "fair balance" of benefit and risk information. For broadcast (radio and TV) only the major side effects must be mentioned and the ads must give a source for additional information, such as a website or the location of a print ad. Most ads are product-claim ads, but the FDA categories help to explain why ads sometimes appear without any information on what the drug is or what it is meant to treat.

DTC advertising of prescription drugs, while prohibited in most of the rest of the world, is big business in the United States. DTC drug advertising is regulated by the FDA, but not in a way that prevents millions from being exposed to ads that the FDA finds misleading. Ads for some drugs are repeated frequently, but only a small number of available drugs are advertised to consumers. There is evidence that DTC advertising contributes to increased drug use and to increased profits, but there is widespread disagreement about whether such advertising serves public health and the public interest. The fact that DTC advertising of prescription drugs is legally permitted in the United States provides no guidance to best ethical practices. There is a clear need to continue to try to understand the consequences and effects, intended and unintended, of DTC advertising.

The last chapter discussed in general terms what the pharmaceutical industry owes the public in their dual role as consumers and citizens. This chapter is intended to build on that discussion by considering some of the major concerns about the practice of advertising prescription drugs to the public. This is followed, in the next chapter, by a consideration of some specific strategies used in DTC drug advertising.

EDUCATING AND EMPOWERING CONSUMERS

Advertising has consequences. Both the extent of advertising prescription drugs to the public and the nature of mass media advertising can be expected to have an impact on the practice of medicine and on health. The actual effects may be intended or unintended or both. Indeed, the industry's intended effects—sell more drugs and improve the public's health—are not always compatible. More consumption of medications is not always better; overuse and misuse of medications are, in fact, among the key issues that need to be addressed in order to improve the quality of healthcare in this country. A good place to start the discussion of the effects of DTC advertising is by considering how such advertising affects patient expectations and how these expectations affect patient-doctor interactions.

Proponents of DTC advertising of prescription drugs argue that one of the major health benefits that can result from prescription drug advertising is consumer education. Consumers are made more aware of symptoms to call to the attention of their doctors. They have information about the availability of specific medications that might be appropriate for their treatment and they can talk to their doctors about that medication. Such advertising "empowers consumers with the information they need to take charge of their own health care."[15] In response to the concern that patients may demand prescriptions for medications that are not appropriate for them, proponents respond that advertising, in encouraging patients to ask their doctors about specific drugs, leaves the prescribing decision with the physician: "Direct-to-consumer advertising does not replace the physician-patient relationship; its purpose is rather to encourage an informed discussion between patient and physician."[16]

There is evidence that many patients do ask their physicians about specific drugs. And, in doing so, they are increasing their chances of getting the drug. According to the FDA survey of patients and doctors, published in 2004: 85% of physicians reported "that their patients asked about prescription drugs frequently." "About half of the patients reported that the doctor prescribed the drug they had asked *about*." Patients "who asked specifically about a particular brand were more likely to receive a prescription for the requested drug than those who had simply asked about whether there was a prescription treatment available for them."[17] The mere fact that it is the physician who writes the prescriptions does not mean, of course, that the decision is always based primarily on an informed and sound medical judgment. Nor does it mean that patient expectation or a patient's request does not determine the outcome at times. It is often difficult for physicians to "disappoint" patients who present with an expectation of a medication.[18]

John Abramson described the effects of DTC advertising as "disempowering" the doctor-patient relationship:

> From my perspective as a family doctor, I found the request for specific drugs deleterious to both the process and content of good doctoring. Once a patient made a request for a specific drug, the success of the visit from the patient's point of view became defined by whether or not the drug was prescribed. At that point, it became hard to recoup the full potential of the encounter. I was less able to broaden discussion beyond the use (or not) of the latest drugs to more effective ways to control symptoms and preserve health.[19]

As was noted in the earlier discussions of marketing as "education," it is important to recognize that selling and education are two different undertakings, involving two different types of communication and two different understandings of desired outcomes. While consumers may learn something from advertising, the information is a means to the goal of selling. As such, it is likely to be incomplete. The pharmaceutical industry is a marketing-driven industry, not an educational organization. The primary purpose of commercial advertising is to increase sales. Increasing sales and providing information may coincide at times, but advertising is not a mechanism for doing real education.

There are two separate but related points here. One, discussed more fully later in this chapter, is that techniques of contemporary mass media advertising are designed to elicit a particular action, not to inform. The methods of advertising are designed to sell products, not provide unbiased information. The second point is that drug companies have a conflict of interest in regard to educating the public about the drugs they sell.[20] Given their commercial goals, it is not reasonable to expect that they have the kind of objectivity that is essential for true education, even if advertising techniques permitted such an approach. Industry representatives might say that the purpose of DTC advertising is "to encourage an informed discussion between patient and physician," but selling through mass media advertising and educating are conflicting interests.

It is worth repeating that the conflict between education and advertising does not mean that consumers do not gain any knowledge at all through drug company ads. They often do. And the information they gain, along with information they acquire from other sources, sometimes enriches their interactions with physicians and leads to improved healthcare. The information that drug companies provide is the kind of information that relates to their promotional goals, however, not to the goal of truly empowering consumers.

> Researchers from Dartmouth Medical School found that only 13 percent of drug ads in magazines used data to describe drug benefits; the remaining 87 percent relied on vague statements. Not a single ad in the study mentioned the cost of the drug. Only 27 percent of ads presented the cause of or risk factors for the disease, and only 9 percent clarified myths and misperceptions about the disease. The positive effects of lifestyle change were mentioned in less than 25 percent of the ads and fewer than three out of ten acknowledged that other treatments were available. Two out of five attempted to medicalize ordinary life issues. (Routine hair loss or a runny nose, for example, became a medical problem requiring treatment with expensive prescription drugs.)[21]

Consumer education on diseases and on available medications can only be done well when separated from the conflicting goals and interests of advertising. Such education would include information about other diseases or conditions in addition to the chronic ones which provide the biggest market for drug companies. It would include information on alternative methods of responding to symptoms and the benefits and risks associated with each. It would include information on comparative costs. Public health agencies and health educators are better positioned to provide the "scientifically based, useful information that will stimulate better conversations between doctors and patients and lead to true empowerment."[22]

IMPLICIT MESSAGES OF DTC ADS

Advertising is a method of informing the public of available products. It is also, and this is more important when considering advertising ethics, a method of creating demand for the products. There has been a growing recognition in recent years that good advertising ethics requires a consideration of the kinds of values or attitudes or expectations or wants that are being promoted or reinforced in advertising. Advertising has both explicit and implicit content.

> In addition to encouraging persons to buy Brand X, many ads have what I term an "implicit content" that consists of messages about, broadly speaking, the consumer lifestyle. This lifestyle consists of a set of beliefs, attitudes, norms, expectations, and aspirations. . . . While individuals may be aware that they are being sold particular products, the crucial issue is the extent to which they are aware of being "sold" this implicit content.[23]

1. One of the implicit messages of DTC drug advertising is that prescription drugs are just like other products used in our everyday lives.

Some critics of DTC advertising of prescription drugs have suggested that one of the implicit messages found in DTC advertising of prescription drugs is that such drugs are simply something to be chosen and used if they fit your image of how you want to live your life. "[T]hese ads and commercials are helping to transform the medical care system from a professional enterprise focused on the health of people to just another marketplace, like those of fast food, cars, and pop music."[24] By being marketed in the same media used to sell cars, fast food, and shampoo, "prescription drugs have become name-brand commodities, enveloped in the kind of fantasy and desire that surrounds the purchase of lifestyle products."[25]

Consider, for example, the Pfizer ads for Celebrex that used the theme "celebrate" and featured images of attractive and active people. How different was this from ads designed to sell other kinds of products? The explicit content is that Celebrex is a medicine for those who suffer from arthritis. The implicit content is that use of a product like this goes hand in hand with a normal desire to feel young, stay active, and avoid body pains. There is now widespread agreement that COX-2 drugs (like Celebrex) have been overused, widely used in cases where they were not appropriate, a fact described in one article as an example of "medicine fueled by marketing."[26] As will be considered more extensively in the next chapter, some specific advertising strategies—such as offering coupons for a free initial supply of prescription drugs—reinforce the message that drugs are just like non-medical products. The listing of the contraindications and side effects associated with a drug (part of the explicit message) can easily be overshadowed by the implicit message that this is just another product for our everyday living.

2. Another implicit message of DTC drug advertising is that most of us need prescription medicines most of the time.

While one of the implicit messages of DTC ads is that prescription drugs are like other commodities that consumers can choose to improve their lifestyle, another implicit message is a little different. The implied message of all the prescription drug ads taken together is that most of us need medicines most of the time, that taking prescription drugs is an essential part of normal life. There is a pill for every ill and for almost every desire to enhance life—for anxiety, for aging bones, for discolored toenails, for sneezing, for sex (at least for males), for blood pressure, for cholesterol, for pain, for sleep. Pharmaceutical advertising thus reinforces the practice of medical associations to emphasize the extent of disease or the risk for disease. The AHA warns that about 100 million Americans have excessive levels of cholesterol; the National Osteoporosis Foundation says that about 34 million Americans have low bone mass; the American Liver Foundation says that 25 million Americans have liver disease; and on and on.[27] "If all those said to be suffering from some ailment are taken into account, it's estimated that there are more than 1.5 billion sick people in the United States—or five times the population. Assuming one-third are in the 'excellent' health they claim, then two out of every three people you pass on the street are walking around with at least eight different maladies."[28] The public is already prepared for the drug-marketing message that prescription medications are a routine part of life.

The Institute of Medicine describes problems with healthcare quality as problems that include underuse (failure to provide proven effective medicine), overuse (unnecessary interventions or treatment not indicated by symptoms), and misuse (interventions causing preventable complications).[29] Both of the implicit messages of DTC advertising described here—that prescription drugs are consumer commodities and that they are a routine part of life—tend to lead to overuse or misuse; they lead to prescriptions for medications not appropriate in the circumstances. Overuse and misuse result not just from patients making explicit requests for brand-name drugs; they also result from the expectations, often unspoken and found among some physicians as well as among patients, that, of course, drugs should be prescribed. And the drugs that come first to mind are the ones most widely promoted. It is not surprising that the American Public Health Association expressed its concern that advertising prescription drugs to the public "may result in the irrational use of drugs that is detrimental to public health."[30]

THE NATURE OF ADVERTISING

To create the demand for particular products, it is first necessary to convince consumers that they have a "need." One method of creating the sense of need is to get people to feel dissatisfied with the way things are. This method has long been used, for example, in the selling of cosmetics and clothes. B. Earl Puckett, then head of the department store chain Allied Stores Corporation, put it this way many years ago: "It is our job to make women unhappy with what they have."[31] If people are happy with the way their hair or their clothes look, they are not so likely to buy something to change their appearance. This approach, used in selling many other products as well, is often quite subtle, not explicit. "Madison Avenue had crafted a winning formula to get people to buy products based on their anxieties, fears, and hopes."[32]

Donald Barlett and James Steele trace the practice of selling medicines through an appeal based on fear and anxiety to the selling of Listerine as a cure for bad breath. Advertising Listerine by raising the fear of "halitosis" was a great success for Lambert Pharmacal Company and provided a lesson about what works in advertising. As the advertising industry's journal *Printer's Ink* reflected in a tribute to Milton Feasley, one of the advertising writers for Listerine: "He dealt more with humanity than with merchandise. He wrote advertising dramas rather than business announcements—dramas so common to everyday experience that every reader could easily fit himself into a plot as the hero or culprit of its action."[33]

The purpose of using dramas or images or celebrities or emotion-laden scenarios in advertising is to elicit a particular response from those who see or hear the ad. Tom Beauchamp explained the difference between "persuasion" and "manipulation" in the effort to get others to respond as we want them to respond. We "persuade" others to do what we would like them to do by appealing to their understanding, by presenting the "good reasons for accepting the desired perspective."[34] In persuasion, the methods used are types of explicit rationale or arguments. People are persuaded when they come to realize, now that they see the real picture more clearly, they want to take the elicited action. "The essence of rational persuasion is inducing change by convincing a person through the merit of the reasons put forward."[35]

We "manipulate" others to do what we would like them to do by influencing them through non-rational appeals. Use of emotional appeals, mental associations, indoctrination, misleading suggestions, and peer pressure are some examples of manipulative behavior. In manipulation, the appeal tends to avoid reasons or argument, or it uses incomplete or inaccurate facts or reasons. "Manipulation is an attempt to induce one to believe what is not correct, unsound, or not backed by good reasons."[36] One is led to act in a particular way without being presented a rational argument or by being prevented from seeing the whole picture clearly.

Advertising is usually described as "persuasive," but it frequently makes use of selling methods that are more manipulative than persuasive (using Beauchamp's understanding of the terms). Ads sell products by associating these products with a sense of attractiveness or belonging, with youth, with beauty, with sex or romance, with power, with social prestige—hardly methods that convince through the merits of the reasons. Anyone who watches TV or browses through magazines can do a quick analysis of ads to recognize these appeals. Manipulation is not the same as coercion. People are often able to resist efforts to manipulate them, in advertising and in other parts of their lives. While not every use of manipulative advertising is unethical, some such uses are. It depends on the extent of manipulation, on the precise technique used, and on the type of product that is being promoted.

Prescription drug ads tend to use emotional appeals similar to those used to sell other products: the ad for a drug to treat depression that pictures a very unhappy woman whose husband is protectively holding their child some distance away from her; the well-known professional athlete in an ad for a product to treat "sexual dysfunction"; the smiling woman walking among flowers in an ad for an allergy treatment; the active and youthful-looking post-menopausal woman in an ad for a drug for the prevention of osteoporosis. There is no rational appeal here, no explanation of how the medication works or why it is a safer and more effective approach than alternatives approaches. The methods are manipulative in that they are without reasons or explanation or argument—or even any presentation of facts. There is no "rational persuasion."

Every bit as important as the fact that the pharmaceutical industry has embraced DTC advertising of prescription drugs is its adoption of the same advertising methods used for other products. It is selling drugs, powerful medications, to people by using the very same advertising techniques that are used to sell consumer items to the public. If the advertising of drugs involved the rational approach Beauchamp describes as persuasive, one could make a much stronger case for drug advertising being educational.

But rational persuasion is not the nature of contemporary mass media advertising.

Good, high-quality medical care is based on sound professional judgments. It needs to be rational, based on the best scientific evidence available. The pharmaceutical industry's business is medicine and the industry should be held accountable for contributing to good medical practice. Legitimate questions can be raised about the level of the industry's commitment to good medicine, to rational medicine, when it introduces its medications to the public through the use of advertising methods that so frequently bypass reasoning and evidence in favor of more emotional appeals. Precisely because the emphasis is placed on selling the product by whatever methods work (as long as they stay within the legal boundaries), advertising "can distort the medical realities of safety and effectiveness" and it "drowns out medical science."[37]

Advertising medicines directly to the public through mass media, if it is to be done at all, should adhere to higher standards than those that have come to dominate advertising of consumer products. Medicines are different. It is not good enough simply to have the FDA protect the public from misleading ads, certainly not if the industry wants to claim that advertising educates the public. It is not good enough for the industry to rely upon the fact that doctors are the ones who actually write the prescriptions. The public can and should demand that the industry itself avoid the kinds of advertising techniques that do not fit, ethically, the nature of the rational and scientific process of treating patients with drugs.

"Hey, with Nexium you just don't feel better, you are better," asserts Mr. Naughton, who had previously been featured in Jeep commercials. "And better is better."[1]

12

Direct-to-Consumer Advertising:
Better Is Better

In October 2004, the Prescription Access Litigation Project (PAL) filed a lawsuit under California's Unfair Competition and False Advertising Laws against AstraZeneca. AstraZeneca makes and markets Nexium, a proton pump inhibitor used in the treatment of gastroesophageal reflux disease (GERD), often called acid reflux. PAL litigates against what it considers to be illegal price inflation of prescription drugs. The suit alleges that AstraZeneca engaged in a fraudulent and unlawful campaign to switch consumers from Prilosec (also made by AstraZeneca) to Nexium before the Prilosec patent expired and before much less expensive generic equivalents became available. The suit alleges that AstraZeneca unlawfully extended its hold on the proton pump inhibitor market by

(i) commencing baseless patent infringement litigation against potential competitors, (ii) conducting misleading studies to support claims of the benefits of Nexium or Prilosec, (iii) engaging in unfair and deceptive marketing and promotional tactics including providing inaccurate and incomplete information to physicians and consumers concerning the benefits of Nexium, and (iv) engaging in improper pricing practices to induce drug purchasers to switch from Prilosec to Nexium.[2]

Of particular interest in the Nexium suit, for purposes of this discussion of DTC advertising, is the claim that the marketing and promotional tactics used are part of the problem. Nexium ranked seventh among prescription drugs sold in the United States within three years of being approved by the FDA. And among the prescription drugs advertised to the public, Nexium is the most heavily promoted of all, with an estimated $257 million spent on DTC advertising in 2003.[3] Advertising has an impact. If prescription drugs are to be advertised to the public through the mass media, we need to focus critical attention on the way they are advertised. Some advertising campaigns and tactics are better, ethically, than others. And, as the actor says in a Nexium ad, "better is better."

As was noted in the last chapter, one of the risks associated with mass media advertising of prescription drugs is that they are promoted as though they were just like consumer products when they are, in reality, fundamentally different. The relevant ethical principle is that different kinds of products need to be promoted differently. Some advertising practices that are ethically acceptable in selling other products are not ethically acceptable in selling medicines. Three advertising practices or strategies used in DTC advertising are examined in this chapter, which concludes with a discussion of the need to implement better standards for prescription drug advertising.

INCENTIVE PROGRAMS

It has become more common for prescription drug ads to offer free samples. The line advising people to "ask your doctor if ———— is right for you" is sometimes changed to "ask your doctor if a free sample of ———— is right for you." These offers of free drugs are included, for example, in some of the ads for Cialis (for "erectile dysfunction") and for Prevacid and Nexium (for acid reflux). The free sample is usually good for one week's worth of medication or for one prescription. The consumer takes the free sample certificate (which is attached to magazine ads as a card or can be printed from the website) along with a prescription from a physician to the pharmacist, who fills the prescription and gets reimbursed by the company. Pfizer introduced a variation of the free sample offer when, to celebrate the sixth anniversary of the launching of Viagra in 2004, it began to offer the "Value Card for Viagra." Viagra users can get a free prescription every time they fill or refill six "qualifying prescriptions."[4]

Companies describe these free drugs as samples or trial offers or as a savings opportunity for patients. They look very much, though, like incentive programs in the marketing of other products—like the rebates automobile companies offer and the frequent flyer programs airlines offer. The use of incentive programs is recognized, generally, as an inducement for consumers to make purchases by an appeal to their financial interests. And, like other incentive programs, the purpose of offers of free prescriptions is to encourage someone to make a purchase that they might not otherwise make and to build brand loyalty. It is not at all clear that a free prescription incentive program in marketing drugs to consumers is a good ethical practice. A review of some of the significant differences between the decision to use a particular prescription drug and the decision to make a consumer purchase suggests that it is not.

One difference is that the decision to use a medication is (or should be) a decision made by the healthcare professional; it is not simply or primarily the consumer's choice.

The pharmaceutical industry recognizes this fact, in one sense, in the "ask your doctor if ——— is right for you" phrase. The use of free offer incentives may well be sending an implicit alternative message, however: "tell your doctor that this is what you want." The consumer already has the certificate in pocket or purse and just needs the doctor to write the prescription in order to get the free drug. All DTC advertising of prescription drugs raises the risk of changing the patient-doctor relationship. The free prescription incentive may be particularly dangerous; it is more influential in changing that interaction from seeking the doctor's professional opinion to asking the doctor to sign off on what is already selected.

A second difference between the decision to use a medicine and the decision to buy a consumer product is that medical treatment decisions can be "wrong" in a way that consumer purchases are usually not.

Whether a consumer purchase is a good one or not is determined by whether it meets the purchaser's goals. And it is normally the individual or the family who determines what these goals are. The goals of medicine are not determined by individual consumers or by their families. Rather, the goals of medicine, and its purpose and role, are socially determined over time, based on scientific research and commonly held values. Healthcare professionals have an ethical responsibility not to agree if they are asked to do something that is not medically appropriate. If a treatment decision is not directed toward a legitimate medical goal, it is "wrong medicine."[5] Drug ads say that the medication "is not for everyone." This kind of statement is not found in the marketing of consumer items and highlights the difference. The consumer purchase model is not appropriate for decisions about drug prescriptions; free sample incentive programs are applying the consumer purchase model where it does not fit.

A third difference between prescription decisions and consumer purchases is the difference in cost-related information.

When faced with the offer of a rebate on a car purchase or the offer to acquire frequent flyer miles on a particular airline, the consumer can compare prices and decide whether it makes personal financial sense to take advantage of the offer. It is not easy for consumers to know the cost of drugs, however, except for those that they are already taking and paying for entirely out-of-pocket. Ads do not include information on cost, and doctors usually are not well informed. It is interesting that the pharmaceutical industry markets drugs as though they were consumer items in many ways, but it does not provide information on the cost.

A fourth difference is that most consumer purchases are not made using shared resources, while many prescription drug purchases include some use of insurance.

After the Medicare drug benefit goes into full effect, it will be even more common that drug purchases involve shared financial resources. Because others are much more directly affected by purchases using shared funds, the patient's role includes a citizen's responsibility—to use only what is needed in order to conserve resources to meet the needs of others. Using inducements for individuals that might encourage them to purchase unnecessary products from shared resources is very different from incentives to purchase their own car from personal or family resources. The same Pfizer news release that announced the introduction of the "Value Card for Viagra" that provides the seventh prescription free included the statement that Viagra is "covered by most health plans."[6] Incentives to spend shared resources are not the same, ethically, as incentives to spend one's own money.

These differences between the decision to use optional consumer products and the decision to use medicines have ethical implications. The risks of harmful consequences resulting from the inclusion of incentive programs in DTC advertising of prescription drugs might well lead to the conclusion that an ethically responsible pharmaceutical company would not engage in this practice.

MEDICAL THERAPY OR MEDICAL ENHANCEMENT

The differences between a consumer product and a prescription medicine have important implications for the ethics of advertising prescription medicines, but there is a complicating factor. Medical technology can also sometimes be used to enhance appearance or performance. Patients sometimes interact with physicians in situations which are more appropriately described as consumer purchases than as medical treatment. An obvious example is cosmetic surgery, but there are other kinds of medical interventions, as well, that are not so much the treatment or prevention of disease as the pursuit of a more acceptable or pleasant lifestyle. In these cases, the decision to have a particular intervention done is the consumer's choice to seek an improvement in appearance or performance, not a medical judgment about how to treat or prevent a disease or remedy a health problem.

The difference between therapy/prevention and enhancement is not always perfectly clear because concepts like health and disease are not precisely defined. "Is short stature a disease? Is aging? Is muscular weakness in a seventy-five year old? Is a crooked nose or bulging thighs? Do these conditions become disease if they provoke personal unhappiness?"[7] The tendency to medicalize life expands the use of medicine into areas that have traditionally been considered within the range of the normal. Changes commonly associated with aging, for example, like hormone changes and reduced sexual functioning, have traditionally been considered normal, but are often seen today as something to be "treated."

Despite the difficulty involved in knowing precisely where to draw the line between medical therapy/prevention and other uses of medicine, it is of practical importance to make some distinction of this sort. We need to know the difference between what is medically indicated or medically necessary and what is simply medically possible. We need to be able to make a decision about what is essential medical care and what is not essential (an important decision in allocating limited healthcare resources). We need to make a judgment about which decisions to use medical interventions are patient/consumer choices and which require professional medical judgments. The use of medical interventions for enhancement purposes is an example of a consumer purchase rather than a medical judgment. It requires that the physician make sure that the patient/consumer is informed about any risks associated with the intervention, and the physician's skill is required to implement the decision, but the judgment about whether the intervention is "indicated" is the patient's more than the doctor's. In medical therapy/prevention, the patient has the final decision about whether to accept what the doctor proposes (consent), but does not have the medical competence to make a good judgment about whether a particular intervention is medically appropriate.

When prescription drugs are advertised to the public using the "life enhancement" appeal, the company is sending a mixed message. The fact that the drug requires a prescription is suggesting that the decision about whether the drug is appropriate or not is a medical decision, not a consumer purchase choice. The life enhancement appeal, on the other hand, is sending the opposite message—that use of this drug can improve your life, even if your health is clearly within the normal range. Selling prescription medicines through a life enhancement appeal can contribute to the public understanding that consumers should be able to get whatever prescriptions they want from physicians, an attitude that can undermine the scientific and professional nature of medicine and the patient-physician relationship.

The ads for Viagra, to treat "erectile dysfunction," (ED) serve as an example, though the comments made here might also apply to the other widely promoted ED drugs, Levitra and Cialis. No longer do the Viagra ads use the original approach of featuring an aging pubic figure (Bob Dole). Now, when the ad uses a celebrity, it is much more likely to be a younger man who is an active athlete. The difference is significant. Viagra is not just for those men, especially older men, who have medical conditions that prevent them from having sexual intercourse anymore. Viagra is also for any man who, for whatever reason, doesn't always have an erection when he would like. In a full-page ad in *The New York Times* for Viagra, most of the top half of the page was a colored picture of a young attractive male being nuzzled by a young attractive female in a skimpy top. The words featured in the picture were: "There's no other tablet proven to work better or faster to treat ED." The text immediately below the picture began with the following verbal message: "You can count on VIAGRA. Why? Because it works. In a recent study, the majority of men had an erection in 20 minutes. And one third of men had success in just 14 minutes."[8] The text also included the advice: "Don't wait. Join the 23 million men worldwide that have turned to VIAGRA. Ask your doctor if a free sample is right for you." Readers are told to go to the Viagra website "right now."

Male visitors to viagra.com are encouraged to take a "sexual health quiz for men" and to print out the results before going to their doctor. The quiz consists of five questions, with responses scored from 0–5 in four of them, 1–5 in the other. The highest possible score is 25 and the lowest is 1. When the scores are calculated, we are told that any score under 21 may be a sign of ED. This means that someone who "most of the time" is able to achieve and maintain an erection and have satisfactory sexual intercourse (scoring 4 out of 5 on each item) still falls into the category of "it may mean you have ED."[9] It is an interesting understanding of disease or dysfunction if sexual health means that men, presumably of any age, are *always* able to have satisfactory sex. No wonder so many millions of men are said to have ED. This is a clear example of changing the meaning of what constitutes health as a way of getting patients to ask their doctors for a medication.

A reasonable interpretation of the visual messages as well as of the verbal messages is that Viagra is being promoted as a sexual performance enhancement as well as a medication for men who are truly unable to have erections. The issue here is not so much that companies are advertising and selling products to facilitate or enhance sexual activity. The real problem is that they are advertising in such a way as to present enhancement as medical therapy. The confusion between the two contributes to irrational health-care decision-making, as does the tendency to expand the notion of disease and to medicalize results of normal life developments. It does not contribute to rational medicine to have it both ways: (1) to market drugs as treatment requiring the judgment of a physician that there is a medical condition that needs treatment and is covered by health insurance; and (2) to market drugs though an appeal to a desire many people have to enhance their lives. Rational healthcare should be expected to distinguish between medical treatments, which are the prerogative of physicians, and enhancement decisions, which are the prerogative of consumers (and normally should not be supported out of shared and limited financial resources). ED medications are the example used here, but a similar concern can be raised about a number of other prescription drug ads.

DIRECT-TO-PATIENT ADVERTISING

In 2002, General Electric Healthcare introduced the Patient Channel, a television broadcast service made available to hospitals for patient rooms and waiting areas, seven days a week, 24 hours a day. The service features a series of health education programs, on such topics as asthma, new baby care, cholesterol, cancer, diabetes, osteoporosis, smoking, and stroke. The programs are interspersed with commercial advertisements, mostly for prescription drugs. The sponsoring companies pay the cost of the programming, which is presented free to hospitals. The ads are similar to the ones seen on home TV. Some hospitals have found this network an attractively priced method of providing patient education. Others, however, have decided not to accept the industry "gift" and have taken a strong stand against this approach to patient education. The Patient Channel is sometimes referred to as an "ad delivery system."[10]

The following statement about the Patient Channel can be found under "Benefits for Patients" on the GE website: "Information is available in hospital rooms at the time patients are most interested in learning more about their medical condition."[11] This "timeliness" relates directly to one major concern been raised about bringing ads into patient rooms:

> The Patient Channel is essentially a marketing tool for the nation's pharmaceutical corporations. It was designed to give them access to a captive audience at a time of maximum vulnerability and emotional distress. In the studied euphemisms of the channel's marketing director, Kelly Peterson, the Patient Channel enables drug companies to "directly associate their products with a particular condition in a hospital setting."[12]

Hospitalized patients are likely to be particularly vulnerable to advertising manipulation. The fact that the drug ads are presented in the hospital setting gives patients a sense that the ads are endorsed by healthcare professionals. The patient is directly under the care of a physician and expects, as well, that any health-related educational programming presented in the hospital has been reviewed for medical and educational appropriateness. The setting is a medical one and the atmosphere is professional. Any normal resistance that a consumer is likely to have to commercial advertising is reduced in such a setting. Messages in the hospital carry more medical authority than they do on the TV at home.

One of the reasons for hospital interest in GE's programming is that it is expected to help them meet accrediting requirements for patient education. In 2003, however, Dennis O'Leary, president of the Joint Commission on Accreditation of Healthcare Organizations (JCAHO), indicated that hospitals are expected to provide education that is specific to individual patient needs, not general televised programming. In a letter to General Electric, he indicated further that the Patient Channel might lead patients to confuse promotion with education: "the viewer is not sufficiently alerted to the transition between educational programming and marketing programming."[13] One might go a step further and acknowledge that, given the conflict of interest involved, there is no place at all for having patient in-hospital education provided by companies whose real business is selling their drugs. As Marcia Angell notes, "drug companies are not really in the education business. (If they were, they would *sell* their educational programs, not give them away or pay people to accept them.)"[14]

Commercial Alert, a non-profit organization that addresses concerns about the effects of commercialism in American culture, together with a coalition of healthcare professionals, sent a letter to CEOs of all 60 hospital chains in the United States with more than 2,000 beds. They asked them not to carry the Patient Channel.[15] The appeal was made to professionals and administrators in healthcare because they have a responsibility to provide medical education in a context free from the conflicts of interest that lead to bias. They have a responsibility to ensure that patients are not taken advantage of in the pursuit of commercial interests. It is also important, however, to question whether this particular advertising strategy is compatible with good ethical practices in the pharmaceutical industry. Drug companies are themselves in the healthcare business and they have their own responsibilities to patients and to the integrity of the healthcare system. The concerns raised about this particular marketing venture are serious enough that companies should voluntarily conclude that it is not compatible with what they owe the public.

TOWARD BETTER ADVERTISING STANDARDS

In December 2004, the FDA sent a warning letter to AstraZeneca about the claims made in marketing Crestor (a cholesterol-lowering medication). After some FDA officials were quoted in the news media expressing concerns about the safety of Crestor, AstraZeneca undertook an aggressive advertising campaign, placing full-page ads in newspapers around the country for several days. In these ads, the company made the claim that "the FDA has confidence in the safety and efficacy" of Crestor and that the FDA had "as recently as last Friday confirmed that Crestor is safe and effective." In its letter to AstraZeneca, the FDA said that neither claim is true.[16]

This episode exemplifies the weakness of the present system of relying upon FDA review, after the fact, to protect the public from false or misleading advertising. The ads had already appeared in papers across the country before the FDA letter was received and they seemed to be effective in halting the decline in the use of Crestor.[17] As can be expected in these sorts of cases, the after-the-fact judgment that the ads included false claims did not prevent the company from influencing public perceptions. Using misleading claims can work to increase sales (or, as in this case, prevent decrease in sales) and the after-the-fact judgment does not change this impact.

The company defended its ads by saying that "We believe that our communications are consistent with what has been communicated to us."[18] This may very well be true; AstraZeneca may have believed that they were not in any way presenting misleading information to the public. Companies, however, are not always in a good position to evaluate the ethical quality of their own ads. Their commercial interests can influence their perceptions, just as these interests conflict with their ethical responsibility to avoid any inaccurate or incomplete or otherwise misleading information to the public about the nature of the product or its benefits, safety, or cost.

One way of improving the drug advertising review process is to require prior review by the FDA. Moving the after-the-fact FDA reviews to before-the-fact approval would offer more protection of the public. The FDA does not presently have that authority, however, and even if given it, would likely only be able to address questions about misleading or deceptive advertising. DTC advertising of prescription drugs raises other issues that also need to be addressed in advance of broadcasting new DTC ads.

In the absence of such a change in the FDA's role, and probably even with such a change, the pharmaceutical industry needs to have a more demanding prospective ethics review process for DTC advertising—perhaps guided by a code or a set of clearly stated principles. Codes are not always fully adequate, but they have some benefits. The process of developing such a code requires explicit attention to what is owed the public in prescription drug advertising. And a code accepted industry-wide levels the playing field by having all companies adhere to the same rules; it reduces any competitive advantage that might come to a company that cuts ethical corners while others are trying to adhere to higher standards.

A good "PhRMA Code on Direct-to-Consumer Advertising of Prescription Drugs" would include more than the legally mandated minimum requirements regarding the kinds of claims that can be made about efficacy and safety. It would also address, for example, the implicit messages of ads and the question of offering free prescriptions. The development of such a code would provide the opportunity to move beyond the assumption that whatever is acceptable in other industries is appropriate in promoting medications. It would also be an opportunity to listen to, and possibly learn from, "outsiders" who are independent and who have an educated sensitivity to the potential impact of advertising claims and methods.

An industry truly committed to good ethical practices in marketing to the public can be expected to use external independent consultants in the development of its standards. The independence required is normally found only in reviewers who do not benefit personally from the company's commercial success. In addition, the reviewers need to be able to make candid assessments based on their best ethical judgment, supported by the expectation that such reports will be welcomed and given serious consideration.

The development of a demanding code for DTC advertising is one way in which the industry can respond seriously to the legitimate concerns that are being raised about DTC advertising. Regardless of how it is done, the standards need to be improved. Current DTC advertising of prescription drugs raises far too many concerns to continue without change.

Conclusion

Pharmaceutical industry leaders often emphasize their investment in research and development and describe their enterprise as research-based or research-driven. Critics, on the other hand, point to the large expenditures drug companies make in marketing their medications and refer to the industry as marketing-driven. I have attempted here to introduce a different perspective, exploring what it means to take a consistent ethics-driven or ethics-based approach to marketing prescription drugs.

An ethics-based approach to marketing recognizes that "good marketing" is about more than selling products and increasing market share. It is about more than complying with applicable laws and regulations. Ethical marketing is about fulfilling responsibilities to stakeholders. Marketing prescription medications is not the same as marketing most other products because the risks to stakeholders are different. Good ethics standards need to be industry-specific. And they need to cover all practices that have raised concerns, not merely prohibit a few of the most egregious ones.

Among the major risks to stakeholders associated with common prescription drug marketing practices discussed in this book are these:

(1) That the quality of the healthcare that patients receive will be compromised by physician conflicts of interest resulting from drug marketing practices.
(2) That medical education of both healthcare professionals and the public will be biased by its close relationship to pharmaceutical marketing.
(3) That the professionalism involved in the doctor-patient relationship will be undermined by direct-to-consumer advertising.
(4) That the ability of society to provide needed care for all will be compromised by the unnecessary use of expensive medications promoted by the drug industry.

These risks are different from the risks to stakeholders in most other industries because the healthcare market is different from the market for other products. Ethics standards that are satisfactory for marketing other products do not meet the need here.

An ethics-based approach to marketing prescription drugs means being driven by the responsibility to avoid practices that place stakeholders at unnecessary risk of harm. One response of the pharmaceutical industry to critics of its marketing practices is to point to all the benefits that come from the medications the industry produces. It is true, of course, that prescription drugs frequently contribute to improved health. The mere fact that the pharmaceutical industry produces some good medications does not mean, however, that every practice that the industry engages in meets high ethical standards or that the risks associated with specific marketing practices are necessary or appropriate. There is no reason to assume, for example, that hiring "guest authors" of clinical research articles contributes to better drugs or better use of drugs. There is no reason to assume that the financial support by pharmaceutical companies for continuing medical education or the direct-to-consumer mass advertising of arthritis drugs means better drugs or better use of drugs. When the industry defends specific practices as contributing to better informed professionals and/or a better informed public, their arguments do, of course, merit serious consideration. These claims merit serious consideration, but not uncritical acceptance. When a risk of harm has been identified, the burden of proof is on those who argue that the risk is necessary or acceptable. The issue is not whether the drug industry does any good, but whether particular marketing practices are appropriate.

In an article in *The Hastings Center Report,* Leon Kass wondered about the impact of a generation of conversation about bioethics: "Though originally intended to improve our deeds, the reigning practice in ethics, if truth be told, has, at best, improved our speech."[1] Kass's concern regarding bioethics applies equally to business ethics. Though it has become fashionable in the corporate world to talk about "stakeholders" and about "ethics" and about being "good corporate citizens," it is not clear that this language has changed the reality for the better. How we talk is an important part of understanding what needs to be done, but changing language by itself does not improve practice.

It has been my purpose and intent to contribute to a sustained and focused discussion of the meaning of good ethical standards for the marketing of prescription drugs. This book is designed to provide a framework for understanding the risks associated with prescription drug marketing practices and the reasons why these risks should be eliminated or reduced. This talk has been designed to affect practices and behaviors; it is not enough simply to talk the talk. It is my hope that those for whom this analysis makes sense will demand changes.

Given the focus on clarifying the pharmaceutical industry's responsibilities, I have mostly avoided discussion of additional regulations that might or should be imposed on the industry. This decision should not be taken to mean, however, that it is out of place for the public to seek to address the problems identified here through the imposition of legally binding regulations. The nature of the industry and its impact on the public good may well require some regulatory solutions. This is especially true if the voluntary efforts are clearly inadequate.

Notes

INTRODUCTION

1. "The Drug Industry: An Overdose of Bad News," *The Economist* 374, no. 8418 (19 March 2005): 73.

2. "The Drug Industry: An Overdose of Bad News," 73.

3. Kaiser Family Foundation, "Americans Value the Health Benefits of Prescription Drugs, but Say Drug Makers Put Profits First, New Survey Shows," news release, 25 February 2005, <http://www.kff.org>.

4. John Abramson, *Overdosed America: The Broken Promise of American Medicine* (New York: HarperCollins, 2004), 26.

5. "Conflicts of Interest on COX-2 Panel," news release, Center for Science in the Public Interest, 25 February 2005, <http://www.cspinet.org>.

6. Gardiner Harris and Alex Berenson, "10 Voters on Panel Backing Pain Pills Had Industry Ties," *The New York Times,* 25 February 2005, <http://www.nytimes.com>.

7. Among those that appeared between the middle of 2003 till the end of 2004 are the following: Abramson, *Overdosed America;* Marcia Angell, *The Truth About the Drug Companies: How They Deceive Us and What to Do About It* (New York: Random House, 2004); Jerry Avorn, *Powerful Medicines: The Benefits, Risks, and Costs of Prescription Drugs* (New York: Alfred A. Knopf, 2004); Donald L. Barlett and James B. Steele, *Critical Condition: How Health Care in America Became Big Business—and Bad Medicine* (New York: Doubleday, 2004); Merrill Goozner, *The $800 Million Pill: The Truth Behind the Cost of New Drugs* (Berkeley: University of California Press, 2004); Katherine Greider, *The Big Fix: How the Pharmaceutical Industry Rips Off American Consumers* (New York: Public Affairs, 2003); David Healy, *Let Them Eat Prozac: The Un-*

healthy Relationship Between the Pharmaceutical Industry and Depression (New York: New York University Press, 2004); Jerome P. Kassirer, *On the Take: How Medicine's Complicity with Big Business Can Endanger Your Health* (New York: Oxford University Press, 2005); Sheldon Krimsky, *Science in the Private Interest: Has the Lure of Profits Corrupted Biomedical Research?* (Lanham, Md.: Rowman & Littlefield, 2003).

8. Lynn Sharp Paine, "Children as Consumers: An Ethical Evaluation of Children's Television Advertising," in *Business Ethics for the 21st Century*, ed. David M. Adams and Edward W. Maine (Mountain View, Calif.: Mayfield, 1998), 388.

9. To the best of this author's knowledge as of March 2005.

10. David Blumenthal, "Doctors and Drug Companies," *The New England Journal of Medicine* 351, no. 18 (28 October 2004): 1889.

11. Angell, xviii.

1. ETHICS AND FOR-PROFIT BUSINESS

1. Jay S. Cohen, *Over Dose: The Case Against the Drug Companies* (New York: Jeremy P. Tarcher/Putnam, 2001), 36.

2. Peter Jennings, *Bitter Medicine: Pills, Profit and the Public Health,* American Broadcasting Corp., 29 May 2002.

3. W. Michael Hoffman, "Business and Environmental Ethics," in *Business Ethics for the 21st Century*, ed. David M. Adams and Edward W. Maine (Mountain View, Calif.: Mayfield, 1998), 493.

4. Kenneth Mason, quoted by Joel Makower, *Beyond the Bottom Line* (New York: Simon and Schuster, 1994), 31–32.

5. Ira Jackson and Jane Nelson, "Profit with Principles," *Currency,* 2003, <http://www.ethicalcorp.com> (22 June 2004).

6. *Principles of Stakeholder Management* (Toronto: Clarkson Centre for Business Ethics, 1999), 2.

7. Hoffman, 497.

8. Lynn Sharp Paine, "Children as Consumers: An Ethical Evaluation of Children's Television Advertising," in *Business Ethics for the 21st Century*, ed. David M. Adams and Edward W. Maine (Mountain View, Calif.: Mayfield, 1998), 388.

9. Cohen, 36.

2. THE PHARMACEUTICAL INDUSTRY AND ITS STAKEHOLDERS

1. Arnold S. Relman and Marcia Angell, "America's Other Drug Problem," *The New Republic* (16 December 2002): 27.

2. O. C. Ferrell, John Fraedrich, and Linda Ferrell, *Business Ethics: Ethical Decision Making and Cases,* 6th ed. (Boston: Houghton Mifflin, 2005), 27.

3. *Principles of Stakeholder Management* (Toronto: Clarkson Centre for Business Ethics, 1999), v.

4. *Principles of Stakeholder Management,* 4.

5. *Principles of Stakeholder Management,* 2.

6. Pfizer, <http://www.pfizer.com> (9 November 2004).

7. Merck, "Mission Statement," <http://www.merck.com> (9 November 2004).

8. PhRMA, "Who We Are," <http://www.phrma.org> (9 November 2004).

9. Relman and Angell, 27.

10. Relman and Angell, 27.

3. DRUG COMPANIES AND HEALTHCARE PROFESSIONALS

1. David Blumenthal, "Doctors and Drug Companies," *The New England Journal of Medicine* 351, no. 18 (28 October 2004): 1885.

2. While I frequently use the terms "physicians" and "doctors" for shorthand purposes, they are intended to include other healthcare professionals, whenever other professionals are also involved in the kinds of relationships to industry that are under discussion.

3. Four books that are particularly helpful in describing these issues are John Abramson, *Overdosed America: The Broken Promise of American Medicine* (New York: HarperCollins, 2004); Marcia Angell, *The Truth About the Drug Companies: How They Deceive Us and What to Do About It* (New York: Random House, 2004); Jerry Avorn, *Powerful Medicines: The Benefits, Risks, and Costs of Prescription Drugs* (New York: Alfred A. Knopf, 2004); Jerome P. Kassirer, *On the Take: How Medicine's Complicity with Big Business Can Endanger Your Health* (New York: Oxford University Press, 2005).

4. American College of Physicians, "Physicians and the Pharmaceutical Industry," *Annals of Internal Medicine* 112 (1990): 624–626.

5. AMA Code of Medical Ethics: E-8.061, <http://www.ama-assn.org>.

6. Susan L. Coyle for the Ethics and Human Rights Committee, American College of Physicians-American Society of Internal Medicine, "Physician-Industry Relations. Part 1: Individual Physicians," *Annals of Internal Medicine* 136, no. 5 (5 March 2002): 396.

7. <http://www.nofreelunch.org>.

8. <http://www.nofreelunch.org>.

9. Blumenthal, 1885–1886.

10. Kassirer, 68.

11. Blumenthal, 1887.

12. Avorn, 292.

13. Coyle, 399.

14. PhRMA, "Who We Are," <http://www.phrma.org> (9 November 2004).

15. *The Federal Register* 68, no. 86 (5 May 2003): 23731+.

16. Blumenthal, 1885.

17. Kassirer, 128.

18. Abramson, 176.

19. Kassirer, ch. 5.

20. Abramson, 126.

21. Avorn, 303.

22. Kassirer, 162.

23. Institute of Medicine National Roundtable on Health Care Quality, "The Urgent Need to Improve Health Care Quality," *JAMA* 280, no. 11 (16 September 1998): 1000–1005.

24. Avorn, 335–336.

25. Kirk O. Hanson, "Best Ethical Practices for the Group Purchasing Industry: A Report to the Audit Committee of the Board of Directors of Premier, Inc.," October 2002, <http://www.premierinc.com>.

4. MEDICAL PROFESSIONALISM AND SCIENTIFIC INTEGRITY

1. Marc A. Rodwin, *Medicine, Money, & Morals: Physicians' Conflicts of Interest* (New York: Oxford University Press, 1993), 9.

2. Abigail Zuger, "When Your Doctor Goes to the Beach, You May Get Burned," *The New York Times,* 24 February 2004, <http://www.nytimes.com>.

3. Zuger.

4. Manuel G. Velasquez, *Business Ethics: Concepts and Cases,* 5th ed. (Upper Saddle River, N.J.: Prentice Hall, 2002), 448.

5. Rodwin, 9.

6. Jerome P. Kassirer, *On the Take: How Medicine's Complicity with Big Business Can Endanger Your Health* (New York: Oxford University Press, 2005), 51.

7. David Blumenthal, "Doctors and Drug Companies," *The New England Journal of Medicine* 351, no. 18 (28 October 2004): 1887.

8. Blumenthal, 1887.

9. D. Katz et al., quoted by Blumenthal, 1887.

10. Katharine Greider, *The Big Fix: How the Pharmaceutical Industry Rips Off American Consumers* (New York: Public Affairs, 2003), 65.

11. Sheldon Krimsky, *Science in the Private Interest: Has the Lure of Profits Corrupted Biomedical Research?* (Lanham, Md.: Rowman & Littlefield, 2003), ch. 5.

12. Krimsky, 76.

13. John Abramson, *Overdosed America: The Broken Promise of American Medicine* (New York: HarperCollins, 2004), 91.

14. Krimsky, 77.

15. Krimsky, 78.

16. Krimsky, 78.

17. Abramson, ch. 3.

18. American Academy of Pharmaceutical Physicians, <http://aapp.org>.

19. Kassirer, 158.

20. Kassirer, 166.

21. Marcia Angell, *The Truth About the Drug Companies: How They Deceive Us and What to Do About It* (New York: Random House, 2004), 163.

22. David B. Resnik, "Industry-Sponsored Research: Secrecy versus Corporate Responsibility," *Business and Society Review* 99 (1998): 32.

5. THE INDUSTRY'S CODE

1. Marcia Angell, *The Truth About the Drug Companies: How They Deceive Us and What to Do About It* (New York: Random House, 2004), 132.

2. AMA Code of Medical Ethics: E-8.061, <http://www.ama-assn.org>.

3. Susan L. Coyle for the Ethics and Human Rights Committee, American College of Physicians-American Society of Internal Medicine, "Physician-Industry Relations. Part 1: Individual Physicians," *Annals of Internal Medicine* 136, no. 5 (5 March 2002): 398.

4. The Washington Legal Foundation, quoted by Jerome P. Kassirer, *On the Take: How Medicine's Complicity with Big Business Can Endanger Your Health* (New York: Oxford University Press, 2005), 19.

5. The Pharmaceutical Research and Manufacturers of America, "PhRMA Code on Interactions with Healthcare Professionals," <http://www.phrma.org>. Reprinted with permission.

6. DRUG SAMPLES

1. Katherine Greider, *The Big Fix: How the Pharmaceutical Industry Rips Off American Consumers* (New York: Public Affairs, 2003), 76.

2. F. M. Scherer, "The Pharmaceutical Industry—Prices and Progress," *The New England Journal of Medicine* 351, no. 9 (26 August 2004): 928.

3. E. L. Backer et al., "The Value of Pharmaceutical Representative Visits and Medication Samples in Community-Based Family Practices," *The Journal of Family Practice* 49, no. 9 (September 2000): 817–819.

4. Marcia Angell, *The Truth About the Drug Companies: How They Deceive Us and What to Do About It* (New York: Random House, 2004), 129.

5. Kaiser Family Foundation, "National Survey of Physicians. Part II: Doctors and Prescription Drugs," March 2002, <http://www.kff.org>.

6. AMA Code of Medical Ethics: E-8.061, <http://www.ama-assn.org>.

7. Greider, 76.

8. Susan L. Coyle for the Ethics and Human Rights Committee, American College of Physicians-American Society of Internal Medicine, "Physician-In-

dustry Relations. Part 1: Individual Physicians," *Annals of Internal Medicine* 136, no. 5 (5 March 2002): 398.

9. Fran Hawthorne, *The Merck Druggernaut: The Inside Story of a Pharmaceutical Giant* (Hoboken, N.J.: John Wiley & Sons, 2003), 127.

10. Greider, 76.

11. Robert Pear and James Dao, "States Trying New Tactics to Reduce Spending on Drugs," *The New York Times,* 21 November 2004, <http://www.nytimes.com>.

12. Pfizer, "Medicines to Change the World," *2003 Annual Report.*

13. Arnold S. Relman and Marcia Angell, "America's Other Drug Problem," *The New Republic* (16 December 2002): 34.

14. Pear and Dao.

15. Jerry Avorn, *Powerful Medicines: The Benefits, Risks, and Costs of Prescription Drugs* (New York: Alfred A. Knopf, 2004), 72.

16. Brian L. Strom, "Potential for Conflict of Interest in the Evaluation of Suspected Adverse Drug Reactions," *JAMA* 292, no. 21 (1 December 2004): 2645.

17. Abigail Zuger, "Caution: That Dose May Be Too High," *The New York Times,* 17 September 2002.

18. Avorn, 172.

19. J. M. Westfall, "Personal Use of Drug Samples by Physicians and Office Staff," *JAMA* 278, no. 2 (9 July 1997): 141–143.

20. Food and Drug Administration, "Prescription Drug Marketing Act of 1987; Prescription Drug Amendments of 1992; Policies, Requirements, and Administrative Procedures," *The Federal Register* 64, no. 232 (3 December 1999): 67745.

21. AMA, E-8.061. E-Addendum II, Guideline 1(h).

22. FDA, 67735.

23. Phil B. Fontanarosa et al., "Postmarketing Surveillance—Lack of Vigilance, Lack of Trust," *JAMA* 292, no. 21 (1 December 2004): 2647.

24. Fontanarosa, 2647.

25. Fontanarosa, 2649.

26. Fontanarosa, 2649.

7. MARKETING IS NOT OBJECTIVE EDUCATION

1. Marcia Angell, *The Truth About the Drug Companies: How They Deceive Us and What to Do About It* (New York: Random House, 2004), 135.

2. Jay S. Cohen, *Over Dose: The Case Against the Drug Companies* (New York: Jeremy P. Tarcher/Putnam, 2001), 148.

3. Cohen, 149.

4. Cohen, 148.

5. Angell, 150.

6. John Abramson, *Overdosed America: The Broken Promise of American Medicine* (New York: HarperCollins, 2004), 91.

7. Jerry Avorn, *Powerful Medicines: The Benefits, Risks, and Costs of Prescription Drugs* (New York: Alfred A. Knopf, 2004), 17.

8. Manuel G. Velasquez, *Business Ethics: Concepts and Cases,* 5th ed. (Upper Saddle River, N.J.: Prentice Hall, 2002), 348–349.

9. Angell, 142.

10. Arnold S. Relman and Marcia Angell, "America's Other Drug Problem," *The New Republic* (16 December 2002): 27.

11. Jeffrey M. Drazen and Gregory D. Curfman, "Financial Associations of Authors," *The New England Journal of Medicine* 346, no. 24 (13 June 2002): 1901–1902.

12. Barry Meier, "Contracts Keep Drug Research Out of Reach," *The New York Times,* 29 November 2004, <http://www.nytimes.com>.

13. Gardiner Harris, "F.D.A. Links Drugs to Being Suicidal," *The New York Times,* 14 September 2004, <http://www.nytimes.com>.

14. Meier.

15. Harris.

16. Pilar Villanueva, "Accuracy of Pharmaceutical Advertisements in Medical Journals," *The Lancet* 361 (4 January 2003): 27.

17. Villanueva, 31.

18. Avorn, 269.

8. MEDICAL EDUCATION

1. Arnold S. Relman and Marcia Angell, "America's Other Drug Problem," *The New Republic* (16 December 2002): 34.

2. John Abramson, *Overdosed America: The Broken Promise of American Medicine* (New York: HarperCollins, 2004), 118.

3. Relman and Angell, 34.

4. Alan F. Holmer, "Industry Strongly Supports Continuing Medical Education," *JAMA* 285, no. 15 (18 April 2001): 2012.

5. The pharmaceutical industry was represented on the task force that developed these guidelines.

6. Arnold S. Relman. "Separating Continuing Medical Education from Pharmaceutical Marketing," *JAMA* 285, no. 15 (18 April 2001): 2010.

7. Joseph S. Ross, Peter Lurie, and Sidney M. Wolfe, "Medical Education Services Suppliers: A Threat to Physician Education," *Public Citizen,* 19 July 2000, <http://www.citizen.org>.

8. Holmer, 2013.

9. ACCME, "Standards for Commercial Support," 2004, <http://www.accme.org>.

10. Holmer, 2001.

11. Ross, Lurie, and Wolfe, 8.

12. Holmer, 2013.

13. Quoted by Ross, Lurie, and Wolfe, 8.

14. Joe Torre, executive of an advertising agency, quoted by Jerome P. Kassirer, *On the Take: How Medicine's Complicity with Big Business Can Endanger Your Health* (New York: Oxford University Press, 2005), 92.

15. ACCME, Standard 4.2.

16. Relman, 2011.

17. Relman, 2011.

18. Kassirer, 128.

19. Kassirer, 129.

20. Kassirer, 111.

21. Niteesh K. Choudhry, Henry Thomas Stelfox, and Allan S. Detsky, "Relationships Between Authors of Clinical Practice Guidelines and the Pharmaceutical Industry," *JAMA* 287, no. 5 (6 February 2000): 614.

22. Quoted by Abramson, 147.

23. Kassirer, ch. 6.

24. Abramson, 227.

25. Kassirer, 111.

26. Relman and Angell, 41.

27. Relman and Angell, 34.

9. CLINICAL RESEARCH AND THE LIMITS OF COMMERCIAL INTERESTS

1. Bruce M. Psaty and Drummond Rennie, "Stopping Medical Research to Save Money," *JAMA* 289, no. 16 (23 April 2003): 2130.

2. Psaty and Rennie, 2129.

3. Psaty and Rennie, 2129.

4. Steven E. Nissen et al., "Effect of Antihypertensive Agents on Cardiovascular Events in Patients With Coronary Disease and Normal Blood Pressure," *JAMA* 292, no. 18 (10 November 2004): 2217–2226.

5. Gina Kolata, "'Normal' Blood Pressure May Still Be Too High," *The New York Times*, 10 November 2004.

6. Marilynn Marchione, "Doctors' Ties to Drug Firms Questioned," *The Detroit News*, 17 October 2004.

7. Marchione.

8. Jerry Avorn, *Powerful Medicines: The Benefits, Risks, and Costs of Prescription Drugs* (New York: Alfred A. Knopf, 2004), 214.

9. Thomas Bodenheimer, "Uneasy Alliance: Clinical Investigators and the Pharmaceutical Industry," *The New England Journal of Medicine* 342, no. 20 (18 May 2000): 1539.

10. David Blumenthal, "Academic-Industrial Relationships in the Life Sciences," *The New England Journal of Medicine* 349, no. 25 (18 December 2004): 2455.

11. Justin E. Bekelman, Yan Li, and Cary P. Gross, "Scope and Impact of Financial Conflicts of Interest in Biomedical Research: A Systematic Review," *JAMA* 289, no. 4 (22/29 January 2003): 463.

12. Bekelman, Li, and Gross, 463.

13. Bodenheimer, 1539.

14. Sheldon Krimsky, *Science in the Private Interest: Has the Lure of Profits Corrupted Biomedical Research?* (Lanham, Md.: Rowman & Littlefield, 2003), 148.

15. Krimsky, 149.

16. Blumenthal, 2455; Bodenheimer, 1541–1542.

17. Richard A. Rettig, "The Industrialization of Clinical Research," *Health Affairs* 19, no. 2 (March/April 2000): 129–146.

18. Bodenheimer.

19. John Abramson, *Overdosed America: The Broken Promise of American Medicine* (New York: HarperCollins, 2004), ch. 7; Jerome P. Kassirer, *On the Take: How Medicine's Complicity with Big Business Can Endanger Your Health* (New York: Oxford University Press, 2005), 167.

20. Arnold S. Relman and Marcia Angell, "America's Other Drug Problem," *The New Republic* (16 December 2002): 33.

21. Kassirer, 162.

22. Bodenheimer, 1541.

23. Reported by Abramson, 105–106.

24. Bodenheimer, 1542.

25. Bodenheimer, 1542.

26. Gardiner Harris, "F.D.A. Links Drugs to Being Suicidal," *The New York Times,* 14 September 2004, <http://www.nytimes.com>.

27. Catherine De Angelis et al., "Clinical Trial Registration: A Statement from the International Committee of Medical Journal Editors," *The New England Journal of Medicine* (8 September 2004), <http://www.nejm.org>.

28. Marcia Angell, *The Truth About the Drug Companies: How They Deceive Us and What to Do About It* (New York: Random House, 2004), 163.

29. Abramson, 94.

30. PhRMA, <http://www.phrma.org>.

31. AAMC, <http://www.aamc.org>.

32. De Angelis.

33. De Angelis.

34. De Angelis.

35. PhRMA, <http://www.phrma.org>. Reprinted with permission.

10. CITIZENS AND CONSUMERS

1. Jerry Avorn, *Powerful Medicines: The Benefits, Risks, and Costs of Prescription Drugs* (New York: Alfred A. Knopf, 2004), 338.

2. George W. Bush, quoted by John Abramson, *Overdosed America: The Broken Promise of American Medicine* (New York: HarperCollins, 2004), 53.

3. Abramson, 46.

4. Committee on Quality of Health Care in America, Institute of Medicine, *To Err Is Human* (Washington, D.C.: National Academy Press, 2000).

5. Abramson, 46. "OECD" is the Organization for Economic Cooperation and Development.

6. Donald L. Barlett and James B. Steele, *Critical Condition: How Health Care in America Became Big Business—and Bad Medicine* (New York: Doubleday, 2004), 13.

7. Abramson, 53.

8. Mark Sagoff, "At the Shrine of Our Lady of Fatima, or Why Political Questions Are Not All Economic," in *Business Ethics: Readings and Cases in Corporate Morality,* 3rd ed., ed. W. Michael Hoffman and Robert E. Frederick (New York: McGraw-Hill, 1995), 466.

9. Leonard J. Weber, *Business Ethics in Healthcare: Beyond Compliance* (Bloomington: Indiana University Press, 2001), 37–38.

10. Lawrence J. Schneiderman and Nancy S. Jecker, *Wrong Medicine* (Baltimore: Johns Hopkins University Press, 1995).

11. Institute of Medicine National Roundtable on Health Care Quality, "The Urgent Need to Improve Health Care Quality," *JAMA* 280, no. 11 (16 September 1998): 1000–1005.

12. Sheila M. Rothman and David J. Rothman, *The Pursuit of Perfection* (New York: Pantheon Books, 2003), ix.

13. Marcia Angell, *The Truth About the Drug Companies: How They Deceive Us and What to Do About It* (New York: Random House, 2004), 262.

14. Avorn, 72.

15. Robert Pear, "Americans Relying More on Prescription Drugs, Report Says," *The New York Times,* 3 December 2004, <http://www.nytimes.com>.

16. Barlett and Steele, 55–56.

17. Avorn, 102.

18. Abramson, ch. 3.

19. Avorn, 246.

20. Angell, 241–242.

21. Angell, 241.

22. Robert Pear, "Health Spending at a Record Level," *The New York Times,* 9 January 2004; Angell, 10–13.

23. Angell, ch. 10.

24. Barlett and Steele, 36.

25. Barlett and Steele, 69–73.

26. Pfizer, "Medicines to Change the World." *2003 Annual Report.*

27. Avorn, 232.

28. Avorn, 232.

29. Avorn, 238.

30. Abramson, 33–36.

31. Angell, 262.

32. Avorn, 246.

33. Barlett and Steele, 36.

34. Avorn, 238.

11. DIRECT-TO-CONSUMER ADVERTISING

1. Donald L. Barlett and James B. Steele, *Critical Condition: How Health Care in America Became Big Business—and Bad Medicine* (New York: Doubleday, 2004), 198–199.

2. Associated Press, "Pfizer Pulling Advertising for Celebrex," *The New York Times,* 20 December 2004, <http://www.nytimes.com>.

3. Richard A. Friedman, letter to the editor, *The New York Times,* 21 December 2004, <http://www.nytimes.com>.

4. Francis B. Palumbo and C. Daniel Mullins, "The Development of Direct-to-Consumer Prescription Drug Advertising Regulation," *Food and Drug Law Journal* 57, no. 3 (2002): 431.

5. Kaiser Family Foundation, "Prescription Drug Trends," March 2003, <http://www.kff.org>.

6. National Institute for Health Care Management, "Prescription Drugs and Mass Media Advertising, 2000," November 2001: 8, <http://www.nihcm.org>

7. United States General Accounting Office, "Report to Congressional Requesters. Prescription Drugs: FDA Oversight of Direct-to-Consumer Advertising Has Limitations": 3, <http://www.gao.gov>

8. United States General Accounting Office, 3.

9. Kaiser Family Foundation, "Impact of Direct-to-Consumer Advertising on Prescription Drug Spending," June 2003: 2, <http://www.kff.org>

10. See Sidney M. Wolfe, "Direct-to-Consumer Advertising—Education

or Emotion Promotion?" and Alan F. Holmer, "Direct-to-Consumer Advertising—Strengthening Our Health Care System," *The New England Journal of Medicine* 346, no. 7 (14 February 2002): 524–528.

11. Palumbo and Mullins, 429.

12. United States General Accounting Office, 22.

13. United States General Accounting Office, 21.

14. Palumbo and Mullins, 428.

15. PhRMA, "Direct-to-Consumer Advertising of Prescription Medicines: Myths and Facts," <http://www.phrma.org>.

16. Holmer, 528.

17. Kathryn J. Aikin, John L. Swasy, and Amie C. Braman, "Patient and Physician Attitudes and Behaviors Associated with DTC Promotion of Prescription Drugs—Summary of FDA Survey Research Results," Food and Drug Administration, 19 November 2004: 3, <http://www.fda.gov>.

18. Matthew F. Holland, "Direct-to-Consumer Marketing of Prescription Drugs: Creating Consumer Demand," *JAMA* 281, no. 4 (27 January 1999): 383–384.

19. John Abramson, *Overdosed America: The Broken Promise of American Medicine* (New York: HarperCollins, 2004), 156–157.

20. Arnold S. Relman and Marcia Angell, "America's Other Drug Problem," *The New Republic* (16 December 2002): 36.

21. Abramson, 154.

22. Wolfe, 526.

23. Richard L. Lippke, "Advertising and the Social Conditions of Autonomy," in *Business Ethics for the 21st Century,* ed. David M. Adams and Edward W. Maine (Mountain View, Calif.: Mayfield, 1998), 378.

24. Jerry Avorn, *Powerful Medicines: The Benefits, Risks, and Costs of Prescription Drugs* (New York: Alfred A. Knopf, 2004), 290.

25. Quoted by Abramson, 157.

26. Barry Meier, "Medicine Fueled by Marketing Intensified Trouble for Pain Pills," *The New York Times,* 19 December 2004, <http://www.nytimes.com>.

27. Barlett and Steele, 195–197.

28. Barlett and Steele, 197.

29. Institute of Medicine National Roundtable on Health Care Quality, "The Urgent Need to Improve Health Care Quality," *JAMA* 280, no. 11 (26 September 1998): 1000–1005.

30. The American Public Health Association, "Direct-to-Consumer Prescription Drug Advertising," a resolution adopted in November 1995.

31. Quoted in Leonard J. Weber, "The Ethics of Health Care Advertising," *Michigan Hospitals* 24, no. 12 (December 1988): 32.

32. Barlett and Steele, 203.

33. Milton Feasley, quoted in Barlett and Steele, 202.

34. Tom L. Beauchamp, "Manipulative Advertising," in *Ethical Theory and Business,* 5th ed., ed. Tom L. Beauchamp and Norman E. Bowie (Upper Saddle River, N.J.: Prentice Hall. 1997), 473.

35. Beauchamp, 474.

36. Beauchamp, 475.

37. Meier.

12. DIRECT-TO-CONSUMER ADVERTISING

1. Stuart Elliott and Nat Ives, "The Media Business: Selling Prescription Drugs to the Consumer," *The New York Times,* 12 October 2004.

2. Prescription Access Litigation, <http://www.prescriptionaccess.org>.

3. Stuart Elliott, "The Media Business: Advertising," *The New York Times,* 19 October 2004.

4. Pfizer news release, 14 April 2004, <http://www.pfizer.com>.

5. Lawrence J. Schneiderman and Nancy S. Jecker, *Wrong Medicine* (Baltimore: Johns Hopkins University Press, 1995).

6. Pfizer.

7. Sheila M. Rothman and David J. Rothman, *The Pursuit of Perfection* (New York: Pantheon Books, 2003), xiv.

8. *The New York Times,* 22 December 2004.

9. <http://www.viagra.com>.

10. <http://www.commercialalert.org>.

11. <http://www.gehealthcare.com>.

12. <http://www.commercialalert.org>.

13. Quoted by Marcia Angell, *The Truth About the Drug Companies: How They Deceive Us and What to Do About It* (New York: Random House, 2004), 151.

14. Angell, 151.

15. News release, <http://www.commercialalert.org>.

16. Gardiner Harris, "Federal Drug Agency Calls Ads for the Cholesterol Pill Crestor 'False and Misleading,'" *The New York Times,* 23 December 2004.

17. Harris.

18. Harris.

CONCLUSION

1. Leon Kass, "Practicing Ethics: Where's the Action?" *The Hastings Center Report* 20, no. 1 (January/February 1990): 8.

Index

Abramson, John, 43, 94, 127, 162
academia, 8, 101–102. *See also* research
access issues, 61, 84, 117, 125, 139
accreditation, 113, 178–179
Accreditation Council for Continuing
    Medical Education (ACCME), 108,
    110–113
acid reflux, 170
Activase, 117
activism, 27–28
advance directive movement, 146–147
adverse reactions, 31, 91
advertising: Celebrex ads, 157–158;
    and consumer education, 161–164;
    in doctors' offices, 37; and drug
    prices, 152–153; and enhancements,
    148–149, 174–177; FDA require-
    ments, 150–152; and free samples,
    82; goals of, 166–169; implied mes-
    sages, 164–166, 181; and incentive
    programs, 171–174; industry defense
    of, 183; legal battles, 170–171; and
    medical education, 114; to patients,
    177–179; public impact, 145; spend-
    ing on, 158–159, 171; standards,
    179–181; types of, 159–161
age-related conditions, 175
Allied Stores Corporation, 166
American Academy of Pharmaceutical
    Physicians, 63

American College of Physicians, 38, 84
American Heart Association (AHA),
    117, 165
American Liver Foundation, 165–166
American Medical Association (AMA):
    and clinical trials, 103; ethics guide-
    lines, 41–42; on free samples, 83, 89;
    on gift practices, 39, 68–69, 115; and
    the PhRMA Code, 67
American Public Health Association, 166
American Society on Internal Medicine,
    84
Angell, Marcia: background, 3; on
    clinical research, 127; critique of the
    pharmaceutical industry, 7–8; on
    drug advertising, 179; on drug selec-
    tion, 149, 154; on new drugs, 86; on
    pharmaceuticals as consumer goods,
    31–32
antidepressants, 102, 126
anxiety-based appeals, 167
approval of new drugs, 87–88, 151
Associated Press, 121
Association of American Medical Col-
    leges (AAMC), 128
Association of Medical Colleges, 103
AstraZeneca, 170, 179–180
authorship, 125, 138, 183
autonomy in healthcare, 114, 146–149
Avorn, Jerry, 88, 97, 121

After more than 30 years on the faculty of the University of Detroit Mercy, LEONARD J. WEBER is now an ethics consultant to healthcare organizations. Most recently he published *Business Ethics in Healthcare* (Indiana University Press, 2001).